Soft Tissue Reconstruction for Digital Defects

Editors

SANDEEP J. SEBASTIN
DAVID M.K. TAN

HAND CLINICS

www.hand.theclinics.com

Consulting Editor
KEVIN C. CHUNG

February 2020 • Volume 36 • Number 1

ELSEVIER

1600 John F. Kennedy Boulevard • Suite 1800 • Philadelphia, Pennsylvania, 19103-2899

http://www.theclinics.com

HAND CLINICS Volume 36, Number 1
February 2020 ISSN 0749-0712, ISBN-13: 978-0-323-73294-9

Editor: Lauren Boyle
Developmental Editor: Kristen Helm

Hand Clinics (ISSN 0749-0712) is published quarterly by Elsevier Inc., 360 Park Avenue South, New York, NY 10010-1710. Months of publication are February, May, August, and November. Business and Editorial Offices: 1600 John F. Kennedy Blvd., Ste. 1800, Philadelphia, PA 19103-2899. Customer Service Office: 3251 Riverport Lane, Maryland Heights, MO 63043. Periodicals postage paid at New York, NY and at additional mailing offices. Subscription price is $439.00 per year (domestic individuals), $854.00 per year (domestic institutions), $100.00 per year (domestic students/residents), $501.00 per year (Canadian individuals), $994.00 per year (Canadian institutions), $562.00 per year (international individuals), $994.00 per year (international institutions), $256.00 (international students/residents), and $100.00 (Canadian students/residents). Foreign air speed delivery is included in all *Clinics* subscription prices. All prices are subject to change without notice. **POSTMASTER:** Send address changes to *Hand Clinics*, Elsevier Health Sciences Division, Subscription Customer Service, 3251 Riverport Lane, Maryland Heights, MO 63043. Customer Service (orders, claims, online, change of address): Elsevier Health Sciences Division, Subscription **Customer Service, 3251 Riverport Lane, Maryland Heights, MO 63043. Tel: 1-800-654-2452 (U.S. and Canada); 314-447-8871 (outside U.S. and Canada). Fax: 314-447-8029. E-mail: journalscustomerservice-usa@elsevier.com (for print support); journalsonlinesupport-usa@elsevier.com (for online support)**.

Reprints. For copies of 100 or more of articles in this publication, please contact the Commercial Reprints Department, Elsevier Inc., 360 Park Avenue South, New York, New York 10010-1710. Tel.: 212-633-3874; Fax: 212-633-3820; E-mail: reprints@elsevier.com.

Hand Clinics is covered in *MEDLINE/PubMed (Index Medicus), Current Contents/Clinical Medicine, EMBASE/Excerpta Medica,* and *ISI/BIOMED.*

Contributors

CONSULTING EDITOR

KEVIN C. CHUNG, MD, MS
Charles B. G. de Nancrede Professor of Surgery, Professor of Plastic Surgery and Orthopaedic Surgery, Chief of Hand Surgery, Michigan Medicine, Assistant Dean for Faculty Affairs, Associate Director of Global REACH University of Michigan Medical School, Ann Arbor, Michigan, USA

EDITORS

SANDEEP J. SEBASTIN, MCh (Plastic Surgery), MMed (Surgery), FAMS (Hand Surgery)
Senior Consultant, Department of Hand & Reconstructive Microsurgery, National University Health System, Singapore

DAVID M.K. TAN, MBBS (Singapore), MMed (Surgery)
Senior Consultant and Residency Director, Department of Hand and Reconstructive Microsurgery, National University Hospital, Visiting Consultant, Department of Orthopaedic Surgery, Changi General Hospital, Assistant Professor, Department of Orthopaedic Surgery, Yong Loo Lin School of Medicine, National University of Singapore, Singapore

AUTHORS

GOO HYUN BAEK, MD, PhD
Department of Orthopaedic Surgery, Seoul National University Hospital, Seoul, Republic of Korea

AMEYA BINDU, MCh, DNB (Plastic Surgery)
Senior Resident, Department of Plastic Surgery, B.J. Govt Medical College & Sassoon Hospital, Pune, Maharashtra, India

ALPHONSUS KHIN SZE CHONG, MBBS, MRCS
Associate Professor, Department of Orthopaedic Surgery, Yong Loo Lin School of Medicine, National University of Singapore, Senior Consultant, Hand and Reconstructive Microsurgery, National University Hospital, Singapore, Singapore

KEVIN C. CHUNG, MD, MS
Charles B. G. de Nancrede Professor of Surgery, Professor of Plastic Surgery and Orthopaedic Surgery, Chief of Hand Surgery, Michigan Medicine, Assistant Dean for Faculty Affairs, Associate Director of Global REACH, University of Michigan Medical School, Ann Arbor, Michigan, USA

SOUMEN DAS DE, MBBS (Hons), FRCSEd (Ortho), MPH
Consultant, Department of Hand and Reconstructive Microsurgery, National University Health System, Singapore, Singapore

JARKKO JOKIHAARA, MD, PhD
Associate Professor, Department of Hand Surgery, Tampere University Hospital, Faculty of Medicine and Health Technology, Tampere University, Tampere, Finland

TEEMU KARJALAINEN, MD, PhD
Senior Research Fellow, Department of Epidemiology and Preventive Medicine, School of Public Health and Preventive Medicine, Monash Department of Clinical Epidemiology, Cabrini Hospital, Monash University, Malvern, Australia; Unit Head, Unit of Hand Surgery, Department of Surgery, Central Finland Central Hospital, Jyväskylä, Finland

YOUNG-WOO KIM, MD, PhD
W Institute for Hand and Reconstructive Microsurgery, W Hospital, Daegu, Republic of Korea

AMITABHA LAHIRI, MBBS, FRCS(Edin), FAMS
Department of Hand and Reconstructive Microsurgery, National University Health System, Singapore, Singapore

YOHAN LEE, MD
Department of Orthopaedic Surgery, Seoul National University Boramae Hospital, Seoul, Republic of Korea

YOUNG HO LEE, MD, PhD
Department of Orthopaedic Surgery, Seoul National University Hospital, Seoul, Republic of Korea

JIN XI LIM, MBBS
Associate Consultant, Department of Orthopaedic Surgery, Ng Teng Fong General Hospital, Department of Hand and Reconstructive Microsurgery, National University Health System, Singapore, Singapore

CHENG-HUNG LIN, MD, FACS
Department of Plastic and Reconstructive Surgery, Chang Gung Memorial Hospital, Linkou Medical Center, Taoyuan City, Taiwan

YU-TE LIN, MD, MS, FACS
Department of Plastic and Reconstructive Surgery, Chang Gung Memorial Hospital, Chang Gung University College of Medicine, Keelung City, Taiwan

NIKHIL PANSE, MCh, DNB (Plastic Surgery)
Associate Professor, Department of Plastic Surgery, B.J. Govt Medical College & Sassoon Hospital, Pune, Maharashtra, India

MICHEL SAINT-CYR, MD
Chief, Department of Surgery, Division of Plastic Surgery, Baylor Scott and White, Temple, Texas, USA

BENJAMIN ZHI QIANG SEAH, MBBS
Resident, Department of Hand and Reconstructive Microsurgery, National University Hospital, Singapore, Singapore

SANDEEP J. SEBASTIN, M.Ch (Plastic Surgery), M.Med (Surgery), FAMS (Hand Surgery)
Senior Consultant, Department of Hand & Reconstructive Microsurgery, National University Health System, Singapore

DAVID M.K. TAN, MBBS (Singapore), MMed (Surgery)
Senior Consultant and Residency Director, Department of Hand and Reconstructive Microsurgery, National University Hospital, Visiting Consultant, Department of Orthopaedic Surgery, Changi General Hospital, Assistant Professor, Department of Orthopaedic Surgery, Yong Loo Lin School of Medicine, National University of Singapore, Singapore

RUTH EN SI TAN, MBBS
Department of Hand and Reconstructive Microsurgery, National University Health System, Singapore, Singapore

POI HOON TAY, MBChB
Resident, Department of Hand and Reconstructive Microsurgery, National University Hospital, Singapore, Singapore

VIGNESWARAN VARADHARAJAN, MS
Registrar, Department of Plastic Surgery, Hand, and Reconstructive Microsurgery, Ganga Hospital, Coimbatore, Tamilnadu, India

HARI VENKATRAMANI, MS, MCh(Plast)
Senior Consultant, Department of Plastic Surgery, Hand, and Reconstructive Microsurgery, Ganga Hospital, Coimbatore, Tamilnadu, India

NICHOLAS WEBSTER, MD
Resident, Department of Surgery, Division of Plastic Surgery, Baylor Scott and White, Temple, Texas, USA

SANG-HYUN WOO, MD, PhD
W Institute for Hand and Reconstructive Microsurgery, W Hospital, Daegu, Republic of Korea

CHARLES YUEN YUNG LOH, MBBS, MSc, MS, MRCS
St Andrew's Centre for Burns and Plastic Surgery, Broomfield Hospital, Chelmsford, United Kingdom; Department of Plastic and Reconstructive Surgery, Chang Gung Memorial Hospital, Linkou Medical Center, Taoyuan City, Taiwan

Contents

Preface: Soft Tissue Reconstruction for Digital Defects xi

Sandeep J. Sebastin and David M.K. Tan

Vascular Anatomy of the Hand in Relation to Flaps 1

Ruth En Si Tan and Amitabha Lahiri

The vascular supply of the hand and wrist is derived from the radial and ulnar arteries. This forms a complex network of vessels on the palmar and dorsal surfaces of the hand. Anastomoses and branching patterns of vessels at the level of the carpals, metacarpals, and phalanges form the basis of old and new flap designs. This article provides an overview on the vascular anatomy of the hand and forearm with emphasis on the blood supply to various flaps.

Adipofascial, Transposition, and Rotation Flaps 9

Hari Venkatramani and Vigneswaran Varadharajan

Numerous random pattern skin flaps have been described based on the subdermal vascular network of the digits. These flaps can be divided based on their composition into skin and adipofascial flaps and on their movement into transposition and rotation flaps. These flaps are suitable for small dorsal defects. Adipofascial turnover flap is a robust and pliable flap with minimal donor morbidity, but needs a skin graft. Transposition flaps are raised adjacent to the defect and move sideways into the defect and requires skin grafting of the donor. Rotation flaps are larger and allow linear closure of the secondary defect.

VY Advancement, Thenar Flap, and Cross-finger Flaps 19

Jin Xi Lim and Kevin C. Chung

The VY advancement, thenar flaps, and cross-finger flaps are workhorse flaps used in reconstruction of fingertip defects. They are reliable and simple to raise without need for microvascular dissection. In addition, they usually provide good results in terms of sensibility and range of motion. This article reviews the history, anatomy, and surgical technique of these flaps with a focus on aesthetic refinements with illustrative cases.

Antegrade Flow Digital Artery Flaps 33

Poi Hoon Tay and David M.K. Tan

Antegrade flow digital artery flaps enjoy a reputation for versatility and reliability with a robust vascular pedicle and the capability of resurfacing small to moderate sized defects in virtually any part of the hand. More than five decades of experience and evolution of surgical techniques with this class of intrinsic hand flaps makes this an indispensable part of the hand surgeons armamentarium when it comes to soft tissue reconstruction in the hand. Variant techniques and variable resurfacing indications are described for these class of flaps in this article. The main disadvantage or limitation lies in the need to sacrifice a digital artery.

Retrograde Flow Digital Artery Flaps 47

Benjamin Zhi Qiang Seah, Sandeep J. Sebastin, and Alphonsus Khin Sze Chong

Retrograde flow digital artery flaps are a versatile single-stage option for the coverage of fingertip and dorsal digit defects. There are technical challenges associated with pedicle dissection and preparation. Techniques vary predominantly in the vessel utilized (either the proper digital artery or its branches) and the incorporation of the digital nerve or its branches in the pedicle with subsequent neurorrhaphy. Venous failure is more common. There is often mild but perceivable donor site morbidity. Evidence favors an innervated flap for better sensory recovery. Cold intolerance follows sacrifice of a digital artery.

Flaps Based on Perforators of the Digital Artery 57

Yu-Te Lin, Charles Yuen Yung Loh, and Cheng-Hung Lin

This review article summarizes the various types of digital artery perforator flaps used in digit reconstruction. The indications for use of digital artery perforator flaps and the preferred approach for reconstructing fingertip defects are explained in this article. Recent updates in digital artery perforator anatomy in the finger, techniques for flap harvest, and inset as well as a delayed approach to using digital perforator flaps in finger reconstruction are discussed.

Flaps Based on Palmar Vessels 63

Nikhil Panse and Ameya Bindu

Video content accompanies this article at http://www.hand.theclinics.com.

The glabrous skin of the palm provides the best color and texture match for reconstruction of palmar aspect of fingers following the principle of reconstructing like with like. Few local axial and perforator flaps have been described of the palm for reconstruction of finger defects. This article reviews the various local flaps based on palmar vessels for digital reconstruction and shares the authors' experiences with similar flaps. Indications, clinical applications, surgical anatomy, and operative techniques of different flaps from palmar tissues are discussed. The authors suggest using these flaps for proximal and smaller defects on the palmar aspect of fingers.

Flaps Based on the Dorsal Metacarpal Artery 75

Nicholas Webster and Michel Saint-Cyr

Video content accompanies this article at http://www.hand.theclinics.com.

Dorsal metacarpal artery flaps have evolved with our knowledge of vascular anatomy of the hand. Since the description of the first transposition flap likely based on the first dorsal metacarpal artery in the 1950s until today, the indications and modifications of these flaps have greatly expanded. Reverse flow flaps have allowed coverage of the dorsum of each digit with vascularized tissue with minimal donor site morbidity and harvest of veins, bone, and tendon with them. This article reviews the history, anatomy, indications, and surgical techniques of this class of flaps and its numerous permutations.

Free Flaps for Soft Tissue Reconstruction of Digits 85

Yohan Lee, Sang-Hyun Woo, Young-Woo Kim, Young Ho Lee, and Goo Hyun Baek

Soft tissue reconstruction of the digit is challenging for hand surgeons because it must satisfy both functional and aesthetic requirements. A wide variety of treatment options exist. A free flap can be an alternative solution in some clinical situations. This article has 2 purposes. First, it discusses various considerations for free-flap usage for reconstruction of soft tissue defects of the digits and the available options. Second, it provides more detailed information regarding the 3 commonly used free flaps, namely, the partial toe pulp flap, radial artery superficial palmar branch flap, and arterialized venous flap.

Soft Tissue Coverage of the Digits and Hand 97

Soumen Das De and Sandeep J. Sebastin

There are multiple options available for reconstruction of soft tissue defects of the digits. The main goal of reconstruction is to achieve normal or near-normal mobility. Soft tissue defects can be considered in the following groups: fingertip, nonfingertip, and multiple digits. The choice of reconstruction for fingertip defects depends primarily on the amount of volar skin available. The patient's functional demands and expectations, and the expertise of the surgeon, also determine the reconstructive strategy.

A Review and Meta-analysis of Adverse Events Related to Local Flap Reconstruction for Digital Soft Tissue Defects 107

Teemu Karjalainen and Jarkko Jokihaara

The authors reviewed the current literature to estimate incidence rates for adverse events with pedicled flaps in the hand. The authors identified 241 different studies reporting adverse events for 6693 flaps. The average incidence rate was 5.4% and total or partial loss of flap constituted 65% of all reported complications. Flaps with reverse or perforator-based flow may be more prone to vascular complications compared with flaps with antegrade flow or skin pedicle. The incidence rates were acceptable in all flaps (1%–10%) and thus the flap can be chosen primarily based on considerations other than risk of adverse events.

HAND CLINICS

FORTHCOMING ISSUES

May 2020
Hand Infections
John Fowler and Rick Tosti, *Editors*

August 2020
Health Policy and Advocacy in Hand Surgery
Kevin C. Chung, *Editor*

November 2020
Managing Axial Instability of the Forearm
Julie E. Adams, *Editor*

RECENT ISSUES

November 2019
Global Hand Surgery: Learning and Contributing in Low- and Middle-Income Countries
Kevin C. Chung, *Editor*

August 2019
Current Concepts and Controversies in Scaphoid Fracture Management
Steven L. Moran, *Editor*

May 2019
Revascularization and Replantation in the Hand
Kyle R. Eberlin and Neal C. Chen, *Editors*

Preface
Soft Tissue Reconstruction for Digital Defects

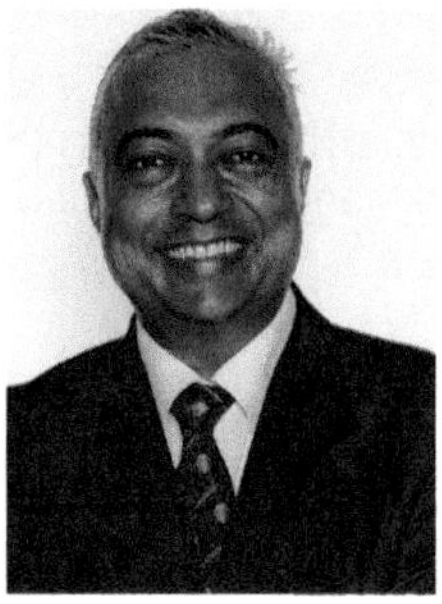

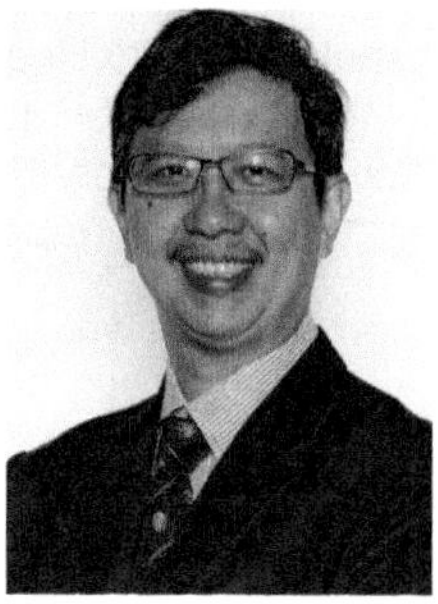

Sandeep J. Sebastin, MCh (Plastic Surgery), MMed (Surgery), FAMS (Hand Surgery)

David M.K. Tan, MBBS (Singapore), MMed (Surgery)

Editors

Soft tissue loss of the hand and digits is a common problem that confronts the hand surgeon and can arise from myriad causes with potential to cause pain, loss of function, and aesthetic disfigurement. The past 5 to 6 decades have seen a steady evolution and invention of different surgical strategies to resurface defects in the digits, ranging from simple single-stage procedures well within the ability of the novice surgeon to complex microsurgical reconstructions feasible in the hands of a practiced microsurgeon. Multiple considerations must be taken into account when deciding on the optimal resurfacing option, not least of which would be the surgical repertoire of the hand surgeon. In fact, the myriad number of flap options in itself can pose a challenge to the beginner.

This issue of the *Hand Clinics* is a compendium of some of the most widely adopted flaps in practice, organizationally bundled according to a functional flap classification. Understanding the blood supply of the hand and within the hand is the key to the safe and successful elevation of any flap. Hence, this issue opens with the article, "Vascular Anatomy of the Hand in Relation to Flaps." The subsequent articles describe and outline different flap options with progressive complexity in ensuing articles. Regardless of the topic covered, every article in this issue is a bountiful repository of knowledge of the described techniques, richly enhanced by a historical perspective, technical pearls and preferences of the authors, and detailed illustrative content. Several articles also stand out for introducing techniques popular among reconstructive surgeons in Asia, including "Flaps Based on Perforators of the Digital Artery," "Flaps Based on Vessels in the Palm," and "Free Flaps for Soft Tissue Reconstruction of Digits." This undoubtedly makes this issue a truly global collection of experience in the field of reconstructive surgery of the hand.

"Considerations in Digital Soft Tissue Reconstruction" and "A Review and Metaanalysis of Adverse Events Related to Local Flap Reconstruction for Digital Soft Tissue Defects" are indispensable reading and neatly round off this issue. The former outlines a schema that the surgeon can use when deciding on the reconstructive options for dealing with singular or multiple soft tissue defects of the hand, and the information from the latter article is something for every surgeon to bear in mind when choosing different flap options.

It has been our privilege to work with many experts of the field in the compilation of this issue, and we are grateful to the contributing authors for the time they have spent in doing research on the topics, sharing their invaluable insights and pearls, and outlining each article in a clear and succinct manner, which should be easy for the reader to assimilate, digest, and translate into practice. We would like to thank the series editor, Dr Kevin Chung, for the opportunity to edit this issue and his contribution of the topical material. We are confident this issue will be a useful

Hand Clin 36 (2020) xi–xii
https://doi.org/10.1016/j.hcl.2019.10.001
0749-0712/20/© 2019 Published by Elsevier Inc.

resource for the reader and gladly welcome any comments or feedback.

Sandeep J. Sebastin, MCh (Plastic Surgery), MMed (Surgery), FAMS (Hand Surgery)
Department of Hand & Reconstructive Microsurgery
National University Health System
Tower Block
Level 11, 1E Kent Ridge Road
Singapore 119228

David M.K. Tan, MBBS (Singapore), MMed (Surgery)
Department of Hand and Reconstructive Microsurgery
National University Hospital
NUHS Tower Block, Level 11, 1E Kent Ridge Road, Singapore 119228

E-mail addresses:
sandeep_sebastin@nuhs.edu.sg (S.J. Sebastin)
david_mk_tan@nuhs.edu.sg (D.M.K. Tan)

Vascular Anatomy of the Hand in Relation to Flaps

Ruth En Si Tan, MBBS, Amitabha Lahiri, MBBS, FRCS(Edin), FAMS*

KEYWORDS

• Vascular anatomy • Upper limb flap • Artery • Circulation • Digit

KEY POINTS

- The radial, ulnar, and interosseous arteries provide the vascular supply of the hand and wrist. The perforators from these vessels form the basis of fasciocutaneous flaps from the forearm that are commonly used in the reconstruction of the hand.
- There are four dorsal metacarpal arteries. The first dorsal metacarpal artery originates from the radial artery, whereas the remaining three originate from the dorsal carpal arch. These continue on the dorsal aspect of the proximal phalanges and communicate with branches of the proper digital arteries at the proximal interphalangeal joints.
- In the hand, the superficial palmar arch forms as the continuation of the ulnar artery (with contribution from the radial artery) and the deep palmar arch as the continuation of the radial artery (with contribution from the ulnar artery). The common digital arteries arise from the superficial palmar arch to supply the fingers and receive contributions from the deep palmar arch. The numerous palmar and dorsal branches of the digital arteries allow for a variety of flaps for digital reconstruction.
- The thumb has two proper digital arteries (radial and ulnar) on the palmar surface that originate from the princeps pollicis artery in most of the population. The dorsal arteries are variable and arise from the first dorsal metacarpal artery. The palmar or the dorsal circulation is sufficient to support the vascularity of the thumb, independent of each other. This allows mobilization of the entire palmar skin as an advancement flap.
- Understanding the blood supply, branches, and perforators to the skin at different levels is important for reconstructive surgery of the hand.

OVERVIEW

The vascular supply of the hand and forearm is a complex network of vessels derived from the radial and ulnar arteries. This typical pattern is observed in 84% of the population. However, there are some variations. There may be a persistent median artery arising from the ulnar artery seen in 8% of the population, or a superficial brachial artery, which is a branch from the brachial artery, present in another 8% of the population.[1]

The radial artery is the smaller of the terminal branches of the brachial artery. It begins in the cubital fossa approximately 2.2 cm inferior to the transverse crease at the level of the neck of the radius.[2] The artery lies within the lateral intermuscular septum of the forearm. Proximally it lies between the supinator muscle and the origin of the flexor digitorum superficialis muscle. In the middle third of the forearm, it lies anterior to the pronator teres. In the distal third it lies anterior to the flexor pollicis longus muscle and ulnar to the tendon of

Disclosure Statement: Neither of the authors has any funding sources, commercial, or financial conflicts of interest to declare.
Department of Hand and Reconstructive Microsurgery, National University Health System, Level 11, Tower Block 1E Kent Ridge Road, Singapore 119228, Singapore
* Corresponding author.
E-mail address: amitabha_lahiri@nuhs.edu.sg

Hand Clin 36 (2020) 1–8
https://doi.org/10.1016/j.hcl.2019.08.001

the flexor carpi radialis tendon. Throughout the proximal two-thirds of its course, it lies posterior to the medial border of the belly of the brachioradialis muscle. The superficial radial nerve runs along with the radial artery in the middle third of the forearm. The radial recurrent artery arises immediately after the origin of the radial artery. It courses proximally superficial to the supinator muscle, and passes anterior to the lateral epicondyle, where it anastomoses with the radial collateral artery, a branch from profunda brachii. Muscle branches supply the muscles on the radial side of the forearm, and septocutaneous branches arise along the entire course of the radial artery. These branches lie within the lateral intermuscular septum. In the proximal two-thirds of the forearm, the lateral intermuscular septum is located between the bellies of the brachioradialis and the flexor carpi radialis. The largest septocutaneous branch is the inferior cubital artery, arising distal to the radial recurrent artery.[2]

Along its course within the lateral intermuscular septum between the brachioradialis and flexor carpi radialis muscles, the radial artery gives rise to multiple periosteal branches to the radius, which allow the harvest of bone segments on the radial artery. Specifically between the insertion of the pronator teres and the brachioradialis muscles on the lateral aspect of the radius, there is no muscle interposed between the radial artery and the radius. At the radiocarpal joint it gives rise to the superficial palmar branch, which joins the superficial branch of the ulnar artery to form the superficial palmar arch. The radial artery then turns around the radiocarpal joint as the dorsal branch, and crosses the anatomic snuff box to the first interosseous space to enter the palm. It then gives rise to the princeps pollicis, the radialis indicis, and terminates as the deep palmar arch.[2]

The ulnar artery is the larger of the two branches of the brachial artery. It passes deep to the heads of the pronator teres and the superficial flexors of the forearm. It then runs in a medial and distal direction anterior to the flexor digitorum profundus muscle. Proximally it is crossed by the median nerve, which passes between the two heads of the pronator teres muscle and courses longitudinally in the midforearm. Immediately after its origin, it gives rise to the anterior and posterior recurrent arteries. Approximately 2 cm from the bifurcation of the brachial artery, it gives rise to a short common interosseous artery that further divides into anterior and posterior interosseous arteries.

In the proximal forearm, the ulnar nerve is lateral to the ulnar artery deep to the muscle belly of the flexor carpi ulnaris muscle. The ulnar artery remains associated to the ulnar nerve throughout the distal two-thirds of the forearm, where it remains on its lateral side.[2]

PERFORATORS FROM THE RADIAL AND ULNAR ARTERIES

The forearm is an ideal donor site for thin fasciocutaneous flaps. There are between 12 and 20 perforating arteries over the radius and ulna. Masquelet[3] and Timmons[4] described that most of the cutaneous branches of the radial artery arise in the distal forearm. Studies by Zbrodowski and colleagues[5] found three to five musculocutaneous branches arising from the radial artery in the proximal third of the forearm, four to six in the middle third, and two to three in the distal third.

In a recent study Kimura and colleagues[6] divided the forearm into 10 zones (10%–100% marked from distal to proximal direction); the highest number of perforators was noted in the distal third of the forearm (labeled 30%) and the next highest concentration was noted in the proximal third in the zone labeled 70%.

The radial artery fasciocutaneous perforators in the distal third of the forearm are the basis for the elevation of the proximally based radial forearm flap. The proximal group of septocutaneous perforators forms the basis of the reverse flow or the distally based radial forearm flap.

The ulnar artery provides vascularity to the skin of the distal two-thirds of the ulnar forearm and the dorsum of the hand. The ulnar artery gives rise to a cutaneous artery 2 to 5 cm before the pisiform. In cadaveric studies by Becker and colleagues[7,8] this cutaneous branch had a diameter of 1 to 1.3 mm and passed dorsally from the ulnar artery deep to the flexor carpi ulnaris muscle. This branch supplied the skin and the fascia (9–20 cm long and 1.5–10 cm wide) over the distal two-thirds of the ulnar side of the forearm. This cutaneous artery forms the basis for the ulnar artery perforator flap, or the Becker flap. Similar to the radial artery the fasciocutaneous perforators in the distal and proximal thirds of the forearm are used as the basis for ulnar artery forearm flap; however, this flap is not preferred because it eliminates the major blood supply of the hand.

THE INTEROSSEOUS ARTERIES

The interosseous arteries arise either from the common interosseous artery, which is a branch of the ulnar artery, or they may arise directly from the ulnar artery. The posterior interosseous artery forms the axis for the posterior interosseous artery faciocutaneous flap. The posterior interosseous artery enters the deep extensor compartment of the forearm, underneath the supinator at an average distance of 7.9 cm from the lateral epicondyle of the humerus. The interosseous recurrent artery originated at this level in 91% of dissected specimens. The posterior interosseous artery gives rise to a series of fasciocutaneous perforators along its length in the septum between the extensor carpi ulnaris and the extensor digiti minimi.[9]

Clinically the axis of the artery is marked as follows. The elbow is flexed 90° and the forearm placed in full pronation. A line drawn from lateral epicondyle to the distal radioulnar joint indicates the axis of the posterior interosseous artery. The cutaneous perforators are found along this line. The average number of posterior interosseous artery cutaneous perforators in the dorsal forearm is 5 ± 2 and most of them are concentrated in the proximal part of the artery.[10]

Three distinct patterns of septocutaneous perforators have been observed: (1) the septocutaneous branches are distributed in two subgroups, one proximal and the other distal, each containing three or four vessels; (2) in the most predominant pattern, multiple small branches arise at 1- to 2-cm intervals along the total length of the posterior interosseous artery; and (3) in the least common pattern, there is a large proximal perforator in the proximal group sharing the same origin as the interosseous recurrent artery, with a larger diameter than the remaining septocutaneous vessels and fanning out into several branches.[9] It anastomoses with the posterior branches of the anterior interosseous artery, forming the anastomotic network on the posterior aspect of the wrist. The anastomosis rate of its terminal and dorsal branch of the anterior interosseous artery is 98.6% to 100%.[11,12]

The anterior interosseous artery courses on the anterior surface of the interosseous membrane. It gives off branches to the radius and ulna and a median branch to the palm. Throughout the forearm, it gives off direct muscle branches and septocutaneous perforators. Usually the proximal septocutaneous perforator is the largest and arises 3 to 4 cm distal to the common interosseous branch. Distally, at the proximal border of the pronator quadratus muscle, the anterior interosseous artery goes to the dorsal side of the interosseous membrane and gives rise to the dorsal septocutaneous branch, which reaches the skin between extensor pollicis longus and brevis, and also gives small branches to extensor muscles and distal radius.[13,14]

THE CARPAL ARCHES

At the level of the carpus the arteries of the forearm communicate to form three dorsal and three palmar arches.

Dorsal Arches

The dorsal radiocarpal arch (**Fig. 1**) lies deep to extensor tendons at the level of the radiocarpal joint. It is present in 80% of the population and receives contributions from the radial artery, the ulnar artery, and a dorsal branch of the anterior interosseous artery in 67% of the population. The dorsal intercarpal arch is consistently seen in all dissections, and lies at the level of the midcarpal joint. It receives contributions from the radial, ulnar, and the anterior interosseous arteries in 60% of the specimens; however, contributions from the radial artery is absent in 20% of specimens and from the ulnar artery in another 20%. The dorsal proximal metacarpal arch is present at the level of the carpometacarpal joints. A complete arch is

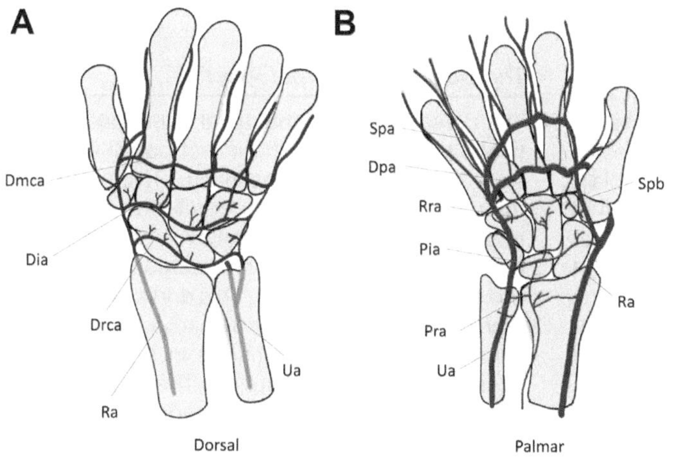

Fig. 1. (*A*) Dorsal and (*B*) palmar blood supply of the carpus. Dia, dorsal intercarpal arch; Dmca, dorsal metacarpal arch; Dpa, deep palmar arch; Drca, dorsal radiocarpal arch; Pia, palmar intercarpal arch; Pra, palmar radiocarpal arch; Ra, radial artery; Rra, recurrent radial artery; Spa, superficial palmar arch; Spb, superficial palmar branch (of radial artery); Ua, ulna artery. (*Modified from* Kuhlmann JN, Guérin-Surville H, Boabighi A. Vascularisation of the carpus, a systematic study. Surg Radiol Anat. 1988;10(1):21-8; with permission.)

seen in 27% of the population. It is supplied by communicating branches of the deep palmar arch.[15,16] This arch gives rise to the second, third, and fourth dorsal metacarpal arteries that supply the dorsal skin of the hand.

Palmar Carpal Arches

There are three palmar carpal arches; the most proximal or the radiocarpal arch is consistently present in 100% of the population. It receives branches from the radial, ulnar, and the anterior interosseous arteries. The palmar intercarpal arch is seen in 53% of the population. Similar to the radiocarpal arch it receives contribution from the three arteries. The distal palmar arch (also known as the distal arterial convergence zone) lies superficial to the bases of the fourth and fifth metacarpals and receives recurrent arteries that are small branches from the radial and ulnar arteries.[15,16]

VASCULAR ANATOMY OF THE HAND

The vascular supply of the hand is derived from the superficial and the deep palmar arches on the palmar aspect and from the dorsal metacarpal arteries that arise from the dorsal metacarpal arch on the dorsal aspect.

THE SUPERFICIAL PALMAR ARCH

The ulnar artery passes through Guyon canal and after giving off a deep palmar branch, which anastomoses with the deep palmar arch (formed predominantly by the radial artery), it continues as the superficial palmar arch that lies superficial to the flexor tendons. At its termination on the radial side of the hand it anastomoses with the superficial palmar branch of the radial artery.

The superficial palmar arch crosses the palm 1 to 2 cm distal to the distal edge of the transverse carpal ligament. The surface anatomy, however, has been a cause of confusion from Kaplan's original drawing where it was depicted at the level of the distal palmar creases. The actual location lies distal to the transverse carpal ligament (**Fig. 2**).[17] It gives rise to the three common digital arteries that divide to form the proper digital arteries of the fingers. The superficial palmar arch is subject to several variations. A complete arch is seen in 42% of cases and is classified as (1) radioulnar (normal), (2) medioulnar (composed of median and ulnar arteries), or (3) radiomedioulnar. The nomenclature is based on the contributing vessels, ulnar artery, median artery, and radial artery.[1] An incomplete arch is seen in 58% of all cases where the common digital arteries arise from ulnar, median, or radial components. Incomplete palmar arches put digits at risk in situations of arterial injuries and when the radial or ulnar arteries have been harvested as parts of a radial forearm or the ulnar forearm flaps.[1]

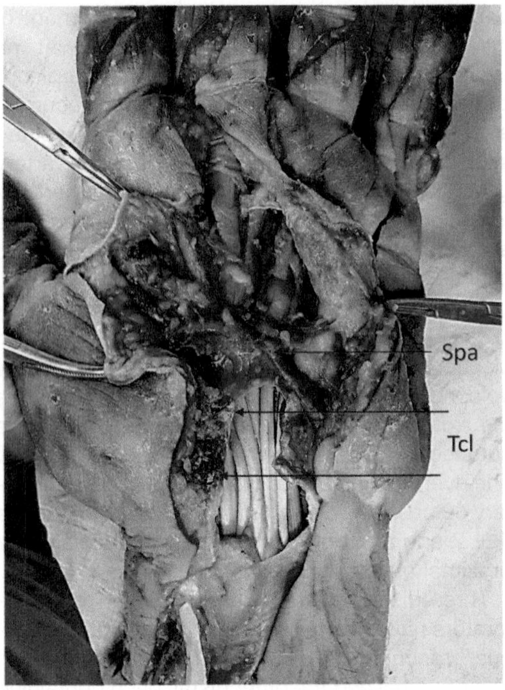

Fig. 2. Location of the superficial palmar arch. Spa, superficial palmar arch; Tcl, transverse carpal ligament (divided) with median nerve excised.

DEEP PALMAR ARCH

The deep palmar arch is the continuation of the dorsal branch of the radial artery. The radial artery enters the palm through the first interosseous space and crosses the palm as the deep palmar arch, lying deep to the flexor tendons. It gives rise to the princeps pollicis artery that supplies the thumb, and branches that communicate with the common digital arteries.

The Dorsal Metacarpal Arteries

The dorsal branch of the radial artery passes between the two heads of the first dorsal interosseous muscle to enter the palm. Before passing through this muscle, it gives rise to the first dorsal metacarpal artery and a transverse branch, which forms the dorsal arch of the carpus (the dorsal proximal metacarpal arch). This dorsal metacarpal arch gives rise to the second, third, and fourth dorsal metacarpal arteries that lie in the respective interosseous regions (**Fig. 3**). The dorsal metacarpal arteries continue on the dorsal aspect of the proximal phalanges and communicate with

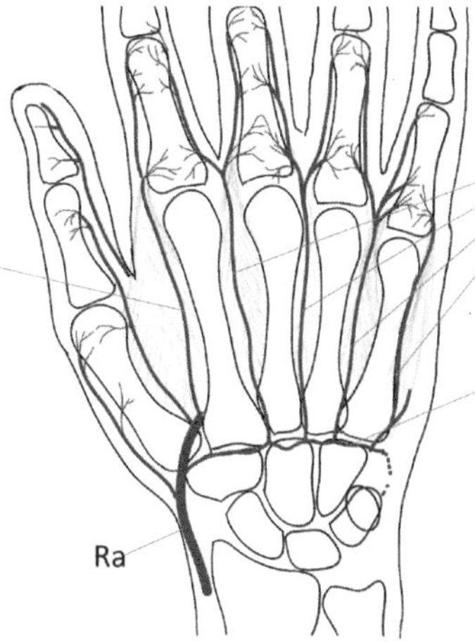

Fig. 3. Dorsal arterial system of the hand. Dma, dorsal metacarpal arteries; Dmca, dorsal metacarpal arch; Fdma, first dorsal metacarpal artery; Ra, radial artery. (*Adapted from* Quaba A, Davison P. The distally-based dorsal hand flap. Br J Plast Surg. 1990;43(1):28-39; with permission.)

the branches of palmar arteries at the level of the proximal interphalangeal joints.

The first dorsal metacarpal artery, which arises directly from the deep branch of the radial artery, is consistent and is the pedicle for the so-called "kite flap." The other dorsal metacarpal arteries connect with the deep palmar network at the level of the metacarpal neck. These interosseous communications form the basis of the distally based dorsal hand flap or the Quaba flap.[18,19] Note that these dorsal metacarpal arteries progressively decrease in caliber and constancy from the radial to the ulnar side of the hand (**Fig. 4**).

VASCULAR ANATOMY OF THE FINGERS (EXCLUDING THE THUMB)

The proper digital arteries arise as the branches of common digital arteries. The neurovascular bundles of each digit are distributed radially from the center of the palm.[20] The ulnar digital artery is larger in the index and middle fingers and the radial vessel is almost always larger in the ring and small fingers. The common digital vessel to the third web space divides into branches that are large on both sides of the web space.[21,22] In some individuals the digital arteries may arise from the deep palmar arch instead of the superficial palmar arch.[23] This may limit the mobility of flaps but does not preclude its use.

PALMAR BRANCHES OF THE DIGITAL ARTERIES

The palmar subcutaneous tissue is vascularized from palmar branches arising from the proper digital arteries. These branches anastomose with their counterparts within the subcutaneous tissue.[24]

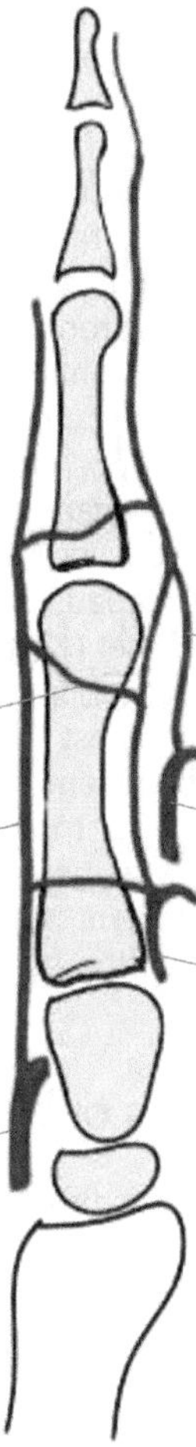

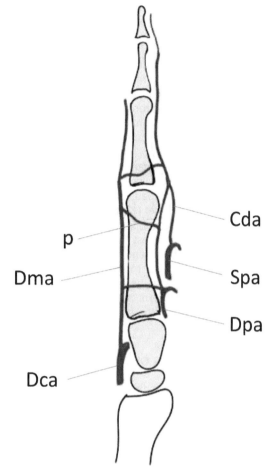

Fig. 4. Dorsal perforators from the deep and superficial palmar systems according to Quaba and Davison. Cda, common digital artery; Dca, dorsal carpal arch; Dma, dorsal metacarpal artery; Dpa, deep palmar arch; p, perforator from deep palmar circulation; Spa, superficial palmar arch. (*Adapted from* Quaba A, Davison P. The distally-based dorsal hand flap. Br J Plast Surg. 1990;43(1):28-39; with permission.)

The proper digital arteries communicate with each other through three major palmar arches that connect the digital arteries: the proximal, middle, and distal transverse arches. The middle transverse and distal arches are 1.5 times larger than the proximal. Their location is constant: the proximal arch is located in association with the C1 pulley and the middle arch in association with the C3 pulley. These arches lie deep to the flexor tendon. These transverse communications between the digital arteries are the basis for distally based vascular island flaps. The distal arch is formed when both digital arteries turn centrally to join each other, just distal to the insertion of the flexor digitorum profundus tendon.[22]

Cadaveric studies have demonstrated an average of 4 to 12 palmar branches from each digital artery at the level of the proximal and middle phalanges.[22,24] These branches travel in the subcutaneous plane and arborize with corresponding branches from the contralateral digital artery. Three types of anatomic branching patterns were observed: (1) I-shaped, consisting of a single vessel (64%); (2) V-shaped, with a bifurcation immediately after the beginning of the vessel (23%); and (3) Y-shaped, branching off beyond the origin of the vessel (13%). It was also noted that these small arterial branches were lateral to the digital nerve in most (82%) cases.[24] These rich connections between the digital arteries and the soft tissue allow for mobilization of islands of palmar skin along with the vessel, such as neurovascular island flaps, or without mobilization of the arteries, such as the homodigital subcutaneous flap.[24]

DORSAL BRANCHES OF THE DIGITAL ARTERY

The dorsal branches have a regular repetitive pattern at the proximal and middle phalanges (**Fig. 5**). Strauch and de Moura [22] described four vessels: (1) a condylar vessel supplying the condylar area of the metacarpal and proximal phalanx, respectively; (2) a metaphyseal vessel supplying the metaphysis of the proximal and middle phalanx, respectively; (3) dorsal skin vessels; and (4) transverse palmar arch vessels (palmar branches), supplying the proximal and middle palmar arches, respectively. These dorsal branches arising from both proper digital arteries supply the skin over the dorsum of the finger. The dorsal branching vessels originating from the proper digital artery in the middle phalanx of finger are constant. These vessels pass distally and dorsally over the middle phalanx and travel distally and obliquely over the distal interphalangeal joint to anastomose with corresponding vessels from the contralateral side of the finger, forming a superficial arcade. A large vascular network across the midline of the finger is normally present.[25] A similar pattern was also noted for the distal phalanx but with some crucial differences. The dorsal skin vessel, arising just before the distal transverse palmar arch, joins with its counterpart from the other side to form the proximal matrix arch. Thereafter, both digital vessels join with each other forming the distal transverse palmar arch.[22]

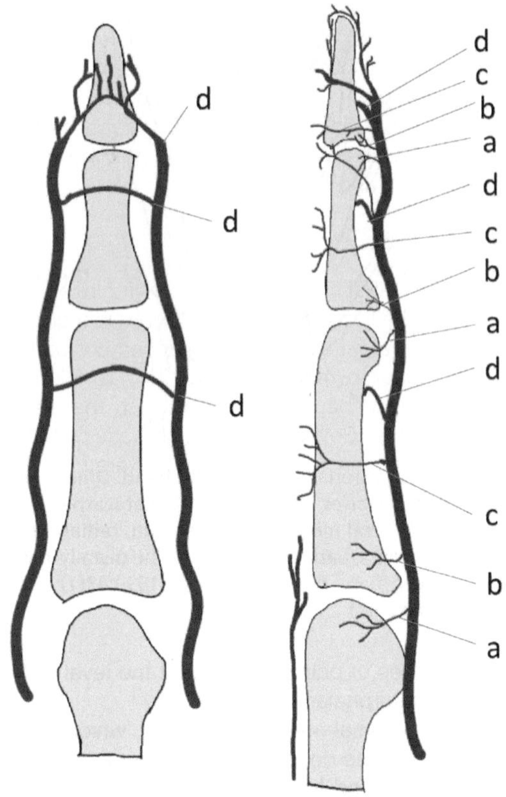

Fig. 5. Branches of the digital artery according to Strauch and Moura. a, condylar vessel; b, metaphyseal vessel; c, dorsal skin vessel; d, transverse palmar arch. (*Adapted from* Strauch B, de Moura W. Arterial system of the fingers. J Hand Surg Am. 1990;15(1):148-154; with permission.)

VASCULAR ANATOMY OF THE PULP AND NAIL BED

Extending from the distal transverse palmar arch are three large vessels that travel to the tip of the pulp and turn dorsally to communicate with the distal matrix arch. There are three dorsal arches that supply the dorsum of the distal phalanx and nail complex, known as the proximal, middle, and distal matrix arches. The two longitudinal lateral vessels on either side of the pulp give off a dorsal branch, which divides into two. Anastomoses from these two divisions form the middle and distal matrix arches, respectively. This branch going dorsally to become the middle and distal matrix arches travels through a defect in the fibrous tissue from the lateral tendon expansion at a point distal to its insertion.[22,25,26]

A network of longitudinal, parallel vessels arising from the distal matrix arch traveling distally gives rise to a superficial capillary network supplying the hyponychium, nail folds, and nail bed. Hasegawa and coworkers[27] observed that within the sterile matrix, there are numerous capillary loops, with the loops becoming longer and more inclined to the nail bed distally. At the level of the germinal matrix, there were no capillary loops. Instead, there was a single layered rectangular plexus of capillaries in the plane of the nail matrix.

VENOUS DRAINAGE OF THE DIGITS

There are two networks of veins: dorsal and palmar. The dorsal system is larger and more constant than the palmar one. Each of these systems resembles a ladder and are interconnected by lateral anastomotic and commissural veins. In a series of dissections, Lucas[28] found a constant vein that terminated over the dorsal midline of the distal phalanx to arborize over the surface of the nail matrix. The veins running longitudinally along the nail margins were also constant. The longitudinal palmar veins do not travel with the arteries. They are situated more superficially and have a more random pattern, traveling in and out of Cleland and Grayson ligaments. In some, there are deep longitudinal veins on the palmar side along the tendon sheath receiving branches from the vincular system.[28]

VASCULAR ANATOMY OF THE THUMB

The thumb has two arterial systems, the palmar and the dorsal systems (**Fig. 6**), either of which is sufficient to support the vascularity of the distal thumb independent of the other.

PALMAR ARTERIES OF THE THUMB

There are two proper digital arteries on the palmar surface: the ulnar digital artery and the radial digital artery. In 90% of individuals, the radial digital artery originates from the princeps pollicis artery and travels radial to the flexor pollicis longus. In 10% of all cases, it is seen to originate directly from the superficial palmar branch of the radial artery.

The ulnar digital artery is larger in diameter and its origin is variable. In 50% to 70% of cases, it originates from the princeps pollicis artery and passes superficial to the insertion of the adductor pollicis. In the other 50% of the population, it may arise from the superficial palmar arch, the superficial branch of the radial artery, or the first dorsal metacarpal artery.[21]

DORSAL ARTERIES OF THE THUMB

The thumb has a dorsal radial and a dorsal ulnar artery. The origin of these dorsal arteries of the thumb is variable.[29] Typically they arise from the first dorsal metacarpal artery, which itself is a branch of the dorsal branch of the radial artery before it enters the palm. The dorsal radial artery arises at the anatomic snuffbox, courses along the abductor pollicis brevis, and terminates as the dorsal arcade at the nail matrix. The dorsal ulnar artery originates either from the first dorsal metacarpal artery or as direct branches from the dorsal branch of the radial artery. Rarely they may originate from the princeps pollicis artery. These arteries are absent in 30% of the population. The robust dorsal vasculature of the thumb allows for mobilization of the entire volar skin on the palmar vasculature as in the Moberg flap without compromising the vascularity of the dorsal skin.[21] The dorsal ulnar artery of the thumb is used to create a distally based island flap for the coverage of thumb pulp defects, also known as the Brunelli flap.[29–31] Likewise the dorsal radial artery of the thumb has been used to design a distally based flap known as the Moschella flap.

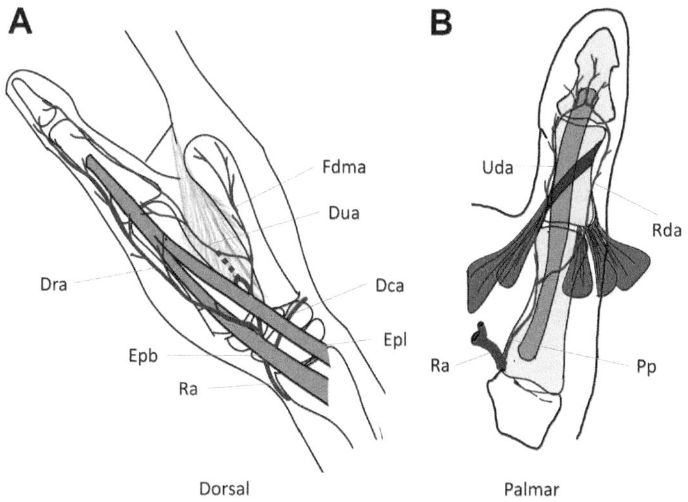

Fig. 6. (*A*) Dorsal and (*B*) palmar arteries of the thumb. Dca, dorsal carpal arch; Dra, dorsoradial artery; Dua, dorsoulnar artery, origin from Fdma or the radial artery (*dotted line*); Epb, extensor pollicis brevis; Epl, extensor pollicis longus; Fdma, first dorsal metacarpal artery; Pp, princeps pollicis; Ra, radial artery; Rda, radial digital artery; Uda, ulnar digital artery. (*Adapted from* Earley MJ. The arterial supply of the thumb, first web and index finger and its surgical application. J Hand Surg Br. 1986 Jun;11(2):163-74.)

SUMMARY

The understanding of the vascular anatomy of the hand and particular awareness of the common variations is crucial for the surgeon performing reconstructive surgery of the hand. Of particular importance are the variations in the communication between the radial and the ulnar systems in the palm. The possibility of incomplete arches must be kept in mind when sacrificing a major vessel for reconstruction. Clinical or Doppler confirmation must be performed before such procedures. Similar caution must be extended to flaps based on digital arteries and possible insufficiency of one of the vessels may compromise the viability of the digit. Besides congenital variations, prior use or shunting of vessels for arteriovenous fistulas for procedures, such as dialysis, must be checked. In other cases, the presence of vasculopathies, such as in diabetes, may compromise the soft tissue circulation and the vessels may be insufficient to support the digit or the flap.

REFERENCES

1. Lippert H, Pabst R. Arterial variations in man. München (Germany): J.F. Bergmann; 1985.
2. Gordon R, Serafin D. Atlas of microsurgical composite tissue transplantation. Philadelphia: Saunders; 2001. p. 389–401.
3. Masquelet A. Anatomy of the radial forearm flap. Anat Clin 1984;6(3):171–6.
4. Timmons M. The vascular basis of the radial forearm flap. Plast Reconstr Surg 1986;77(1):80.
5. Zbrodowski A, Marty F, Gumener R, et al. Blood supply of the subcutaneous tissue of the upper limb and its importance in the subcutaneous flap. J Hand Surg 1987;12B(2):189–93.
6. Kimura T, Ebisudani S, Osugi I, et al. Anatomical analysis of cutaneous perforator distribution in the forearm. Plast Reconstr Surg Glob Open 2017; 5(10):e1550.
7. Becker C, Gilbert A. The ulnar flap. Handchir Mikrochir Plast Chir 1988;20(4):180–3 [in German].
8. Becker C, Gilbert A. The cubital flap. Ann Chir Main 1988;7(2):136–42 [in French].
9. Costa H, Pinto A, Zenha H. The posterior interosseous flap: a prime technique in hand reconstruction. The experience of 100 anatomical dissections and 102 clinical cases. J Plast Reconstr Aesthet Surg 2007;60(7):740–7.
10. Mei J, Morris S, Ji W, et al. An anatomic study of the dorsal forearm perforator flaps. Surg Radiol Anat 2013;35(8):695–700.
11. Penteado C, Masquelet A, Chevrel J. The anatomic basis of the fascio-cutaneous flap of the posterior interosseous artery. Surg Radiol Anat 1986;8(4):209–15.
12. Zancolli E, Angrigiani C. Posterior interosseous island forearm flap. J Hand Surg Br 1988;13(2):130–5.
13. Martin D, Rivet D, Boileau R, et al. The posterior radial epiphysis free flap: a new donor site. Br J Plast Surg 1989;42(5):499–506.
14. 1Syed S, Zahir K, Zink J, et al. Distal dorsal forearm flap. Ann Plast Surg 1997;38(4):396–403.
15. Freedman D, Botte M, Gelberman R. Vascularity of the carpus. Clin Orthop Relat Res 2001;383:47–59.
16. Gelberman R, Panagis J, Taleisnik J, et al. The arterial anatomy of the human carpus. Part I: the extraosseous vascularity. J Hand Surg Am 1983;8(4): 367–75.
17. Ghee C, Lahiri A, Lim A. A clinically feasible method of surface marking for the superficial palmar arch based on correlation of size-matched angiograms to fixed landmarks in the hand. Plast Reconstr Surg 2010;125(3):123e–4e.
18. Quaba A, Davison P. The distally-based dorsal hand flap. Br J Plast Surg 1990;43(1):28–39.
19. Sebastin SJ, Mendoza RT, Chong AK, et al. Application of the dorsal metacarpal artery perforator flap for resurfacing soft-tissue defects proximal to the fingertip. Plast Reconstr Surg 2011;128(3):166e–78e.
20. O'Brien B. Neurovascular pedicle transfers in the hand. ANZ J Surg 1965;35(1):1–11.
21. Earley MJ. The arterial supply of the thumb, first web and index finger and its surgical application. J Hand Surg Br 1986;11(2):163–74.
22. Strauch B, de Moura W. Arterial system of the fingers. J Hand Surg Am 1990;15(1):148–54.
23. Tubiana R, Duparc J. Restoration of sensibility in the hand by neurovascular skin island transfer. J Bone Joint Surg Br 1961;43-B(3):474–80.
24. Voche P, Merle M. Vascular supply of the palmar subcutaneous tissue of fingers. Br J Plast Surg 1996;49(5):315–8.
25. Flint MH. Some observations on the vascular supply of the nail bed and terminal segments of the finger. Br J Plast Surg 1955;8(3):186–95.
26. Shrewsbury M, Johnson RK. The fascia of the distal phalanx. J Bone Joint Surg Am 1975;57(6):784–8.
27. Hasegawa K, Pereira B, Pho R. The microvasculature of the nail bed, nail matrix, and nail fold of a normal human fingertip. J Hand Surg Am 2001; 26(2):283–90.
28. Lucas GL. The pattern of venous drainage of the digits. J Hand Surg Am 1984;9(3):448.
29. Elliot D, Wilson Y. V-Y advancement of the entire volar soft tissue of the thumb in distal reconstruction. J Hand Surg Br 1993;18(3):399–402.
30. Brunelli F, Vigasio A, Valenti P, et al. Arterial anatomy and clinical application of the dorsoulnar flap of the thumb. J Hand Surg Am 1999;24(4):803–11.
31. Brunelli F, Gilbert A. Vascularization of the thumb. Anatomy and surgical applications. Hand Clin 2001;17(1):123–38.

Adipofascial, Transposition, and Rotation Flaps

Hari Venkatramani, MS, MCh(Plast)*, Vigneswaran Varadharajan, MS

KEYWORDS

• Dorsum finger • Adipofascial flaps • Flap cover • Soft tissue cover • Dorsal vascular anatomy

KEY POINTS

- Adipofascial turnover flap is an excellent option for coverage for dorsal defects of the digits. The flap is based on the constant branches arising from the proper digital artery along the proximal and middle phalanges. It is a robust and pliable flap that can be folded on itself to fill dead spaces with minimal donor site morbidity.
- Transposition flaps are raised adjacent to the defect and moved sideways into the defect to cover it. They may be based distally, proximally, or laterally and typically require skin grafting of the donor site. The finger only allows narrow flaps to be raised.
- Rotation flaps are raised along the side of the defect. The flap uses laxity of the adjoining tissues for tension-free linear closure of the primary as well as the secondary defect. The flap rotates as a semicircle with a point of rotation being adjacent to the defect. Typically this flap is useful for small localized defects, such as those overlying the joint.

INTRODUCTION

Dorsal defects of the digits pose a unique challenge for reconstruction. The skin is thin, and any damage or defects would immediately expose the underlying extensor tendon, bone, and joint. Early soft tissue cover is important to avoid permanent damage to the critical structures beneath.

Anatomy of the finger is unique with thick glabrous skin on the palmar side and thin, pliable skin on the dorsum. There is an elaborate network of vessels crossing over from each side of the proper digital artery to the back of the digit. Numerous local skin flaps have been described based on this vascular network. These flaps can be divided based on their movement into transposition and rotation flaps and on their composition into skin and adipofascial flaps. Local flaps like transposition, rotation, and perforator-based local flaps provide stability but lack the mobility and pliability features of adipofascial flaps.

A layer of adipofascial tissue lies between the dorsal skin and the extensor tendons, containing the dorsal veins within. This layer is the basis of an adipofascial flap. It is a flexible layer that can be folded to add bulk and fill dead spaces. The vascular basis of this flap is the branches of the proper digital artery and its anastomoses with the dorsal metacarpal system. These flaps can be designed as proximally based, distally based, or laterally based. These flaps need to be covered with a skin graft, and the excellent vascularity usually results in good take of the graft. The other advantage of this flap is the minimal donor site morbidity as compared with regular skin flap.

Disclosures: None.
Department of Plastic Surgery, Hand, and Reconstructive Microsurgery, Ganga Hospital, 313, Mettupalayam Road, Coimbatore 641043, Tamilnadu, India
* Corresponding author.
E-mail address: drhariv@gmail.com
Twitter: @harimicro (H.V.)

Hand Clin 36 (2020) 9–18
https://doi.org/10.1016/j.hcl.2019.08.002

The design of transposition and rotation flaps on the finger usually requires some modification to the classical design because the fingers are cylindrical compared with the flat surfaces over the trunk, limbs, or the face. Longitudinal defects exposing tendons or bones can be covered with a long unipedicled transposition flap or a bipedicled straplike flaps from uninjured sides. However, these flaps need skin grafting for the donor defects. Small circular defects around the joints can be easily covered by rotation flaps.

HISTORICAL PERSPECTIVE

Hynes[1] in 1954 showed that deepithelialized skin, when turned upside down, will readily take as a free graft. Ivan Pakiam[2] in 1973 applied the same principle and used reverse dermis flaps to cover defects over dorsum of digits, ankle joint, dorsum of the foot, and even a deltopectoral defect following a forelimb avulsion. Erdogan Atasoy[3] in 1978 has been using the same principle to reconstruct full-thickness dorsal skin defects with reverse cross finger flaps. Thatte and colleagues[4] in 1982 also used these turnover flaps to cover defects over the palmar aspect of the fingers. The formations of epithelial cysts, as a result of buried hair follicles, were seen following the use of deepithelialized skin which has led to the modification in 1991 by Lai,[5] who used random pattern adipofascial turnover flaps without deepithelializing. Most of these flaps were designed to cover semicircular or ovoid defects. Yii and Elliot[6] described the homodigital bipedicle strap flap that used the uninjured dorsolateral tissues of the digits to cover longitudinal defects over the dorsum of digits.

The classical description of dorsal digital arteries running longitudinally and supplying the skin over the dorsum of proximal phalanx seen in older anatomic texts was challenged by Levame and colleagues[7] in 1967. They proposed that the proper digital arteries give rise to obliquely running branches supplying the entire length of the dorsal skin of the fingers. Based on these findings, Smith in 1982 described an obliquely oriented sliding flap to cover the dorsal skin defects.[8]

Numerous studies came up in the second half of the twentieth century describing the dorsal arterial system.[9–11] In 1990, Strauch and de Moura[12] proposed that the dorsal skin vessels are constantly present, branching from the proper digital artery. They concluded that the skin over the dorsum of each phalanx has the potential to be used as a pedicled flap. Braga-Silva and colleagues[13,14] established that there were 2 constant dorsal branches that originated from the proper digital artery in the proximal and middle phalanx at fixed distances from the proximal interphalangeal joint. Vuppalapati and colleagues[15] in 2004, through their clinical and cadaveric studies, highlighted the utility of the reverse dorsal digital artery flap to cover more distal defects on the dorsum of fingers.

INDICATIONS AND CONTRAINDICATIONS

Indications:

- Defects over dorsum of the fingers extending from the metacarpophalangeal joint to the tip of the fingers up to 20 × 10 mm in size
- Exposed joints
- Mid lateral defects
- Complete or partial pulp loss

Contraindications:

- Underlying comminuted fractures of the phalanges
- Fingers with compromised vascularity
- Partial degloving injuries
- Smokers

VASCULAR ANATOMY

On the dorsum of the finger, the extensor tendon lies closely opposed to the bone. Overlying the tendon is a vascularized layer of paratenon. Between the paratenon and dorsal skin lies a highly vascular and pliable adipofascial layer. This layer provides a gliding surface and is supplied by well-defined dorsal branches from the proper digital artery at specified intervals.

The vasculature of the dorsum of the fingers can be divided into 3 zones as suggested by Endo and colleagues.[16] The terminal branch of the dorsal metacarpal artery and the dorsal branches of the proper digital artery form the source vessels. The 3 zones are as follows:

1. The region over the web and the metacarpal head.

   Two dorsal digital arteries arise from the dorsal metacarpal artery, one for each adjacent digit, at the level of metacarpophalangeal joint. These arteries join the proximal dorsal branch of the proper digital artery at the midportion of the proximal phalanx.
2. The dorsum of the proximal phalanx.

   The proper digital artery gives rise to the proximal dorsal branch at the midpoint of the proximal phalanx just distal to the proximal finger crease. The size of the proximal dorsal branch is 0.3 to 0.6 mm. A distal dorsal branch arises from the proximal digital palmar arch, at the neck of the proximal phalanx.

3. The dorsum of the middle phalanx.
   The proximal dorsal branch in this region arises from the proper digital artery at the level of the proximal third of the middle phalanx. The size of this artery is 0.3 to 0.5 mm. The distal dorsal branch arises from the distal digital palmar arch that is formed by an anastomosis between the radial and ulnar proper digital arteries. The distal dorsal branch gives rise to 2 notable branches, one forming an arch over the nail matrix and the other supplying the skin over the distal interphalangeal joint.

Strauch and de Moura[12] studied the arterial system of the fingers in 141 human cadavers. According to them, the branches of the proper digital artery followed a consistent branching pattern in the proximal and middle phalanx. Each proper digital artery has a condylar branch, a metaphyseal branch, a dorsal skin branch, and the transverse palmar arch. The proximal and middle phalanx has a proximal and distal transverse palmar arch in close relation to the C1 and C3 cruciate pulleys, respectively. This pattern becomes a complex one in the distal phalanx, where there are proximal, middle, and distal nail matrix arches (**Fig. 1**). In summary, there are 2 groups of dorsal branches arising from the proper digital artery, arranged proximal and distal to the proximal interphalangeal joint.

In a cadaver study of 144 fingers, Braga-Silva and colleagues[14] showed that the vascular system of the dorsum of the finger consisted of 3 dorsal branches of the proper digital artery over the proximal phalanx and 2 over the middle phalanx. The first dorsal branch over the proximal phalanx was inconsistent.[14] The second dorsal cutaneous branch was consistently present 10 mm proximal to the proximal interphalangeal joint in all fingers. The mean diameter of this branch at its origin was 0.3 mm. The third dorsal cutaneous branch lies 4 mm proximal to the proximal interphalangeal joint. The 2 dorsal cutaneous branches over the middle phalanx lie 7 and 12 mm distal to the proximal interphalangeal joint, respectively. They concluded that defects in the middle and distal phalanges could be covered with flaps based on these dorsal cutaneous branches.

Flaps raised in close proximity to the nail fold must ensure the preservation of branches arising from the digital arteries approximately 10 mm proximal to the eponychial fold. Delia and colleagues[17] showed that dissection distal to this point would hamper the vascular supply of the flap. Earlier Strauch and de Moura,[12] have also stressed that the branch traveling from the middle transverse palmar arch, up to meet the proximal matrix arch, must be taken into account, in order to better preserve the vascularity of the skin.[12]

ADIPOFASCIAL FLAPS

Two types of adipofascial flaps have been described in the literature to cover the dorsal digital defects. The random type adipofascial turnover flap described by Lai and colleagues[18] is harvested from the dorsum of the injured digit and has its base along the edge of the defect. The flap can be used as a heterodigital or homodigital turnover flap and is safe as long as a length-to-breadth ratio of 1:1.5 is maintained. A pedicled type adipofascial turnover flap, described by Voche and Merle,[19] is based laterally on one of the dorsal branches of the proper digital artery (**Fig. 2**).

Surgical Technique

This flap is raised under tourniquet control. The wound over the dorsum of the finger is debrided thoroughly in 3 dimensions. The depth of the wounds especially over the joints is visualized and washed. If the joint is exposed and unstable or there is loss of central slip, a K-wire is used to stabilize the joint in extension. Any nonviable and undermined edges should be opened up, and the overlying skin is retained because the flap will fill the cavity. The flap is designed to be always

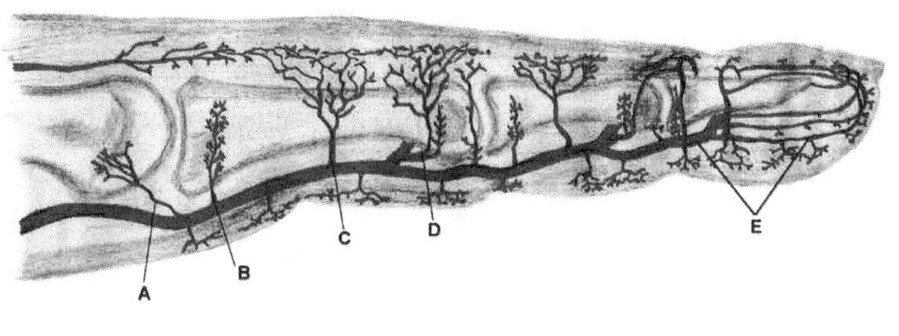

A, Condylar vessel; B, Metaphyseal vessel; C, Dorsal skin vessel; D, Transverse palmar arch; E, Nail matrix arches

Fig. 1. Vascular anatomy of the finger showing branches of the vessel.

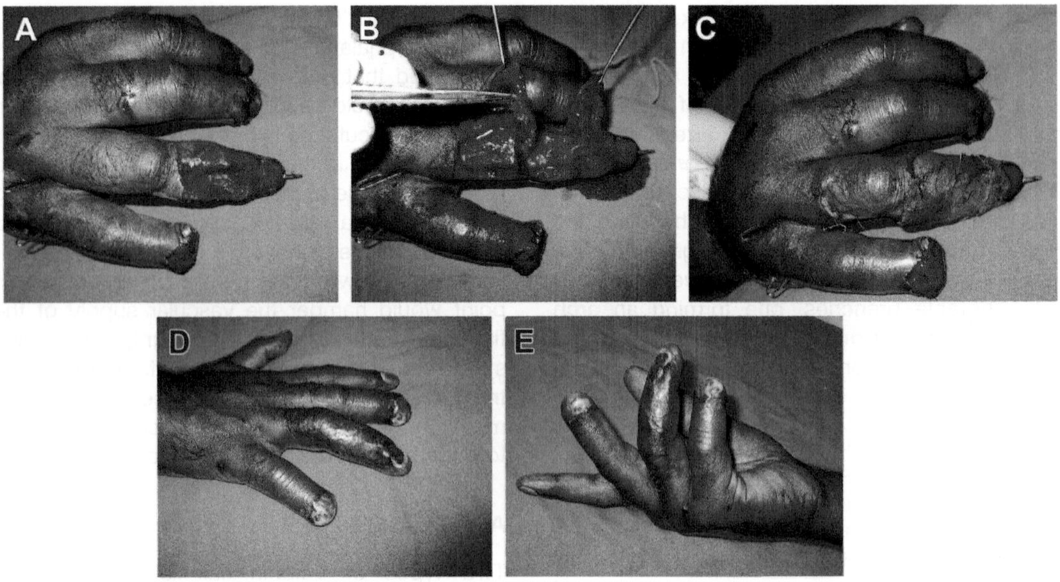

Fig. 2. (*A*) Defect showing the dorsal composite loss of right ring finger. (*B*) Adipofascial turnover flap raised based on the vessels along the edge of the defect being turned over. (*C*) Flap inset into the defect covered with skin graft. (*D, E*) One year postoperative follow-up showing complete healing.

more than the size of the defect in order to fill the cavity and the undermined edges. The length-to-breadth ratio of the flap is generally 1:1.5 if elevated as a random pattern flap and as 1:2, when elevated based on one of the dorsal branches of the proper digital artery proper (**Fig. 3**).

The initial skin incision can be made along the midlateral line or in the midline. The authors prefer the midlateral incision to avoid the adherence of the extensor tendons to the overlying suture line, which is encountered with dorsal midline incisions. The midlateral incision also allows the scar to be relatively concealed. In addition, exposure of critical structures following skin necrosis at the suture line can be avoided. A dermal thickness skin flap is raised below the level of hair follicles, leaving the dorsal vein uninjured in the bed. The adipofascial flap is then raised dividing the veins along the edges. The flap is raised superficial to the extensor tendon taking care to leave the paratenon intact, as done in the case of a classic cross finger flap. The flap is dissected until the pedicle is visualized and turned over to cover the defect (**Fig. 4**). For a wider defect, the flap is based on the source vessel lying along the lateral margin of the flap. The contralateral margin of the flap is divided, and the flap is transposed, rather than turned over. The transposition allows a greater reach of the flap (**Fig. 5**). It is important to handle this flap in an atraumatic manner. The authors have found that holding the flap with skin hooks instead of forceps reduces the degree of postoperative flap edema.

After flap elevation, the tourniquet is released; the vascularity of the flap is ensured, and hemostasis is achieved. The flap is inset, and the raw surface covered with split skin graft harvested from the ipsilateral forearm. The dermal flap is replaced and secured with 5-0 Prolene sutures. The authors have found that venous drainage and subsequent edema are a problem in adipofascial flaps, especially those with 180° of turnover. However, it will settle down over a period of 7 to 10 days. There may also be small areas of graft loss, but may epithelialize rapidly. When the defect is large, the reach of the flap can be increased by designing it in a curvilinear fashion.

Advantages:

- Simple, reliable, and single-stage procedure
- Pliable and thin; can be turned in any direction
- Minimal donor site morbidity
- Can fill small cavities and dead spaces
- The reach can be extended as per the need and size of the defect
- Sensation develops over a period of time
- Spares the proper digital artery
- Useful in multiple finger defects when traditional options like cross finger flap or neurovascular island flaps are not possible

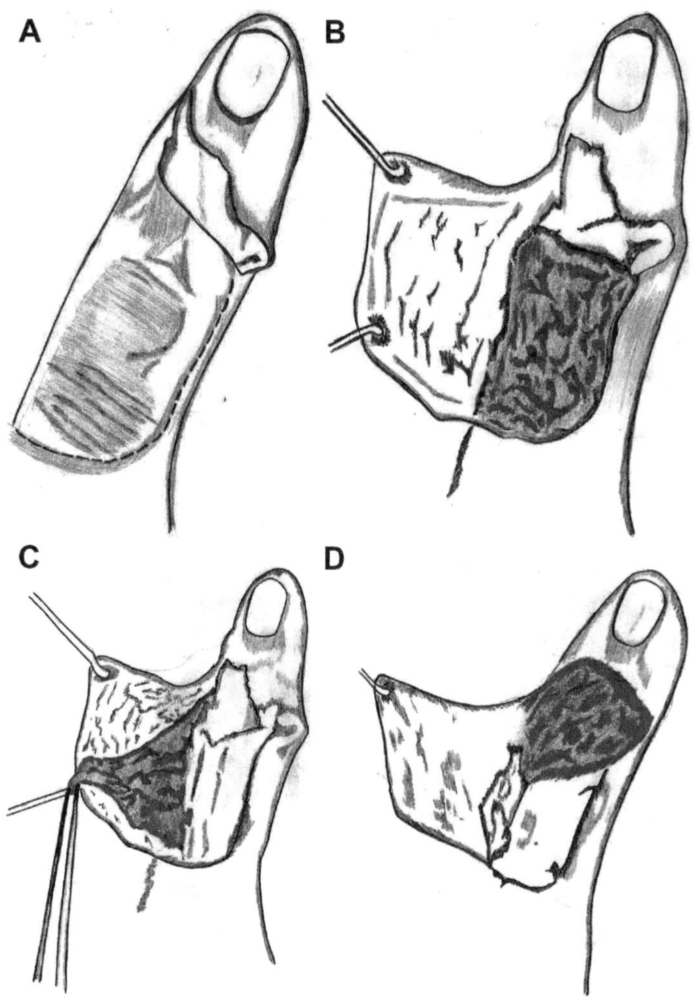

Fig. 3. (*A–D*) Raising of adipofascial flap and transferring it based on names perforator.

- The amount of skin graft required is smaller, as the dermal flap can be replaced

Pitfalls:

- Thinner dermal flaps can cause desquamation and later depigmentation of the replaced skin flap
- Including portions of dermis can lead to epidermal cysts
- Skin grafts need to be of moderate thickness
- Early mobilization to prevent stiffness

TRANSPOSITION FLAP

The design of transposition flaps for dorsal defects of the finger is different from other parts of the body because of the cylindrical shape of the finger (**Fig. 6**). The traditional transposition flap requires triangulation of the defect followed by transposition of the flap. Typically, these flaps cover the primary defect well but require skin graft for the secondary defect.[20] In fingers, the transposition flap can be raised as

- Distally or proximally based
- Laterally based
- Bipedicle

Surgical Technique

Distally or proximally based transposition flap

Surgery is performed under pneumatic tourniquet control and with loupe magnification. Once the defect is created after thorough debridement, a template of the flap is designed based on the size of the defect. The skin flap adjacent to the defect over the dorsum of the same finger is raised superficial to the paratenon, along the midlateral line. In the fingers, the distal extent of the flap has to be designed beyond the defect in order to mitigate the tension generated across the flap

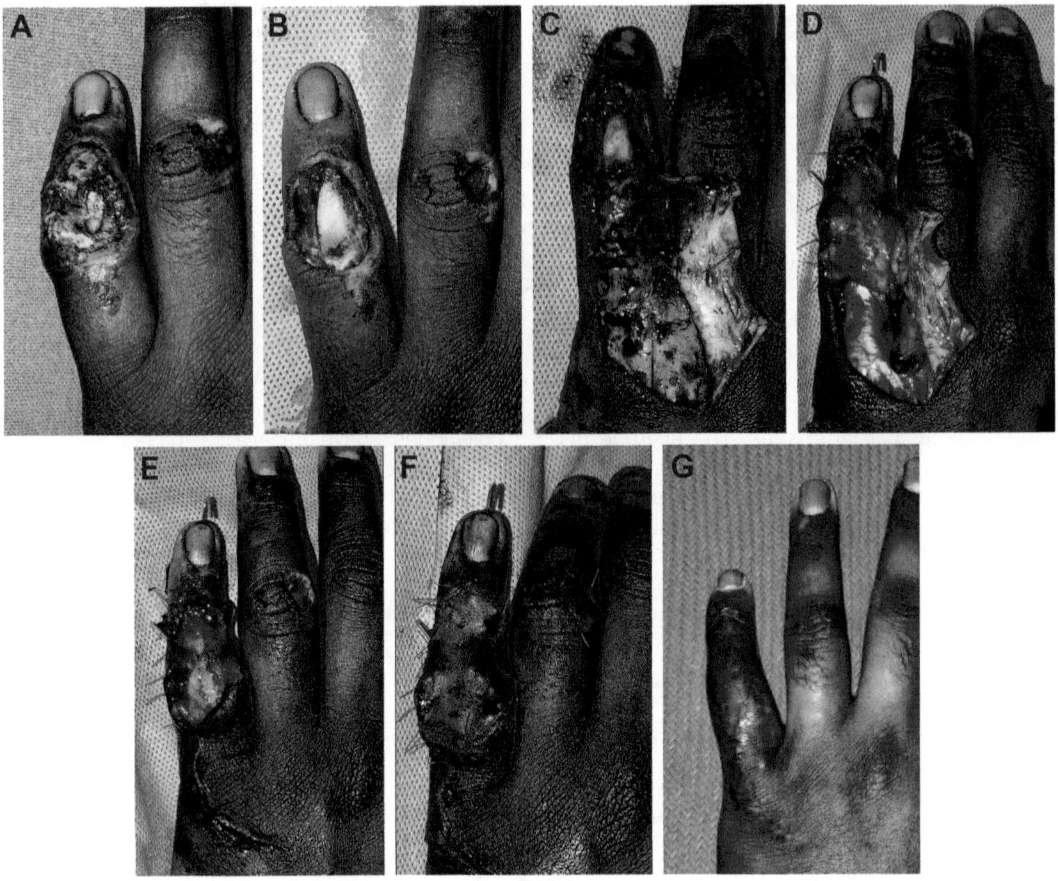

Fig. 4. (*A, B*) Defect overlying middle phalanx of the little finger exposing bone and extensor tendon predebridement and postdebridement. (*C, D*) Adipofascial flap based on the fourth web space dorsal vessels. (*E, F*) Flap inset into defect and covered with skin graft with closure of dermal flap. (*G*) Well-healed flap with settled donor site suture lines.

when the fingers are flexed. The flap is raised with the base proximally or distally and transposed over the defect. The triangular donor defect is skin grafted (**Fig. 7**). When the secondary defect is narrow, resembling a release incision, it can be left alone and allowed to heal by secondary intention.

Laterally based transposition flap

The difference between laterally based and proximally/distally based flaps is that the base is along the midlateral line on 1 side. The flap is broad enough to cover the defect. The pivot point is along the radial or ulnar lateral border of the proximal phalanx (**Fig. 8**). Along the base of the flap, small perforator vessels can be seen.

Advantages:

- Easy to raise
- Longer flaps can be raised with the robust blood supply
- Similar color and texture match
- More stable cover
- Preserved sensation

Disadvantages:

- Limited mobility and area that can be covered
- Can expose the extensor tendon and neurovascular structures
- Requirement of skin grafts for donor area resulting in contour defects

ROTATION FLAP

The flap rotates along the defect, and unlike a transposition flap, it does not have a secondary defect that requires skin grafting. Once the defect is marked on the finger, the flap needs to be designed, keeping the arc in such a way that the diameter is at least 3 to 4 times the diameter of the defect. A common mistake is to raise a smaller flap that is unable to cover the defect without significant tension.

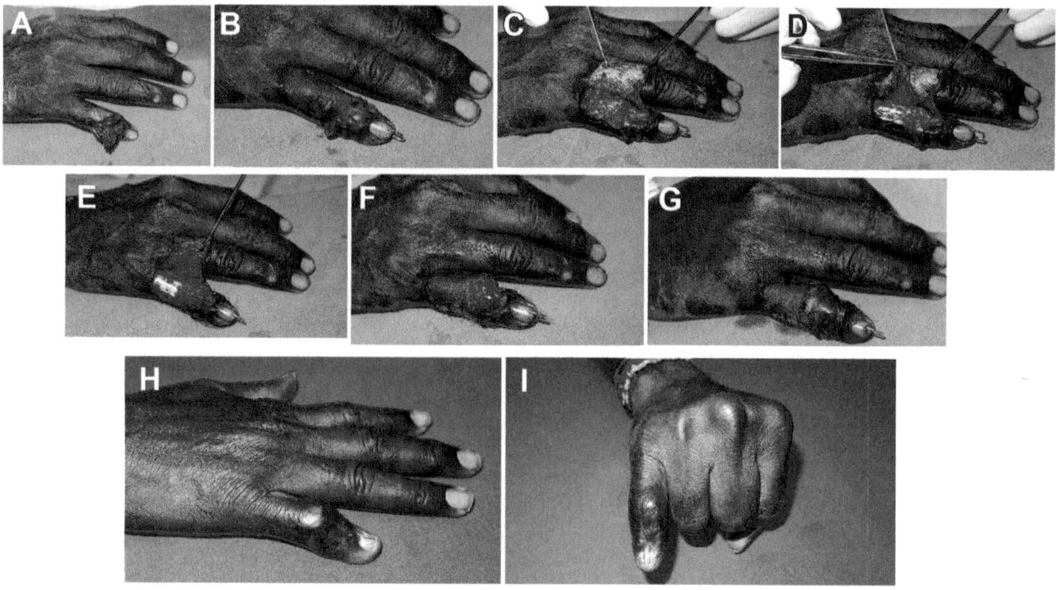

Fig. 5. (*A*) Composite defect with bone and extensor loss over the distal interphalangeal joint. (*B, C*) Design of flap marked with raised dermal flap and adipofascial flap waiting for turnover. (*D, E*) Adipofascial flap based on proximal interphalangeal joint level perforator being folded on itself and filling the cavity. (*F, G*) Flap in situ with closure of dermal defect and split skin graft over the flap. (*H, I*) Long-term outcome showing well-settled flap.

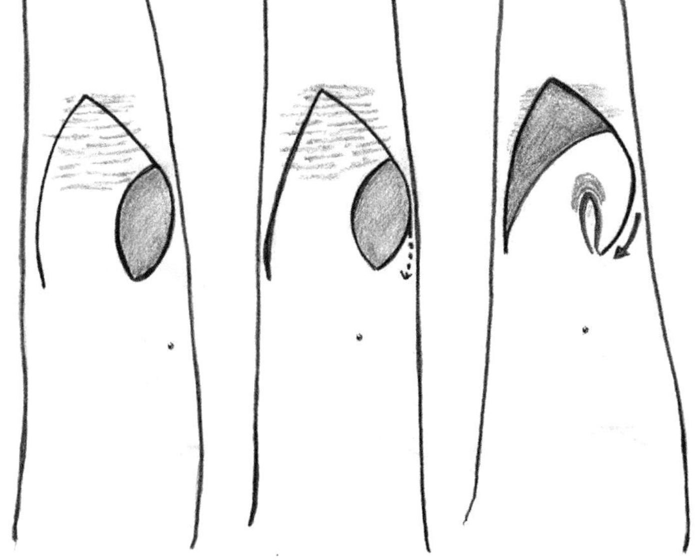

Fig. 6. (*A–C*) Raising of the transposition flap.

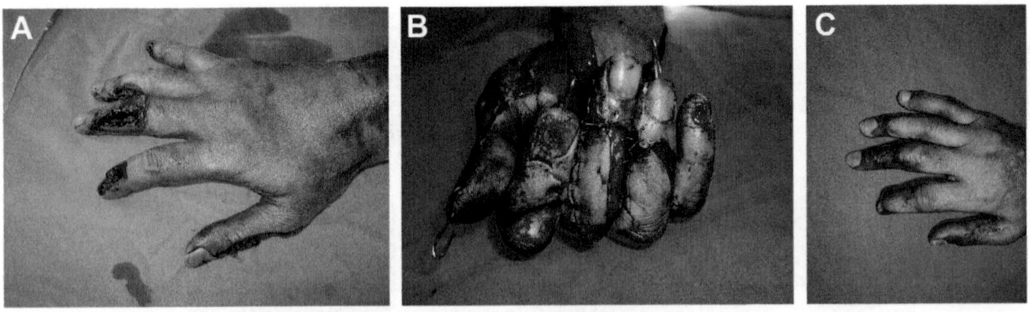

Fig. 7. (*A*) Deep aggressive wound with loss of skin over thumb, index, middle, and ring fingers. (*B*) Transposition flap raised to cover the defects. (*C*) Long-term outcome.

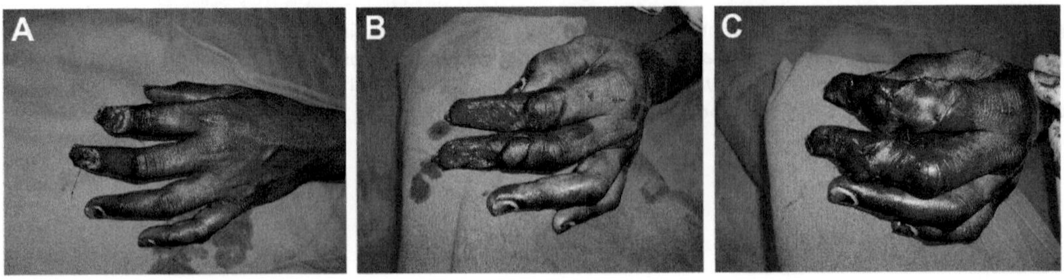

Fig. 8. (*A*) Deep grinding machine injury with loss of nail bed complex and skin. (*B*) Transposition flap marked with base along the sides. (*C*) Flap inset into the critical area with skin graft of donor sites.

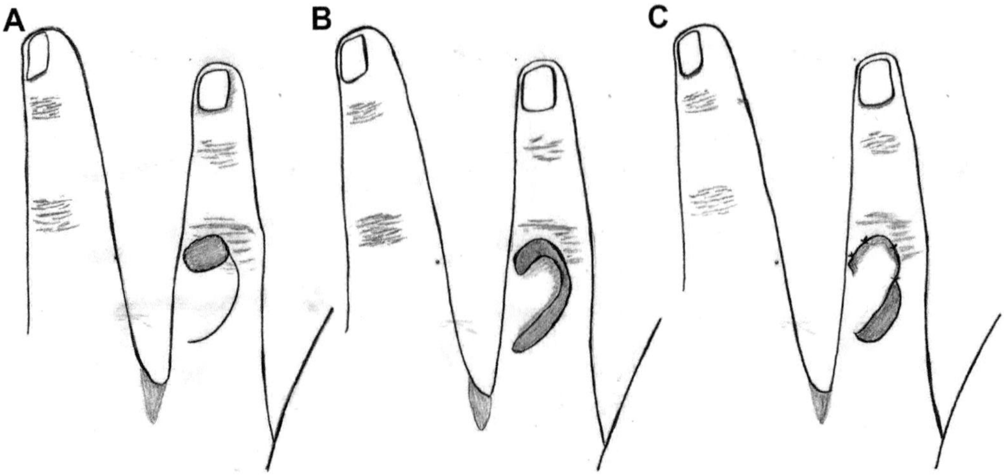

Fig. 9. (*A–C*) Raising of a rotational flap over dorsum of finger.

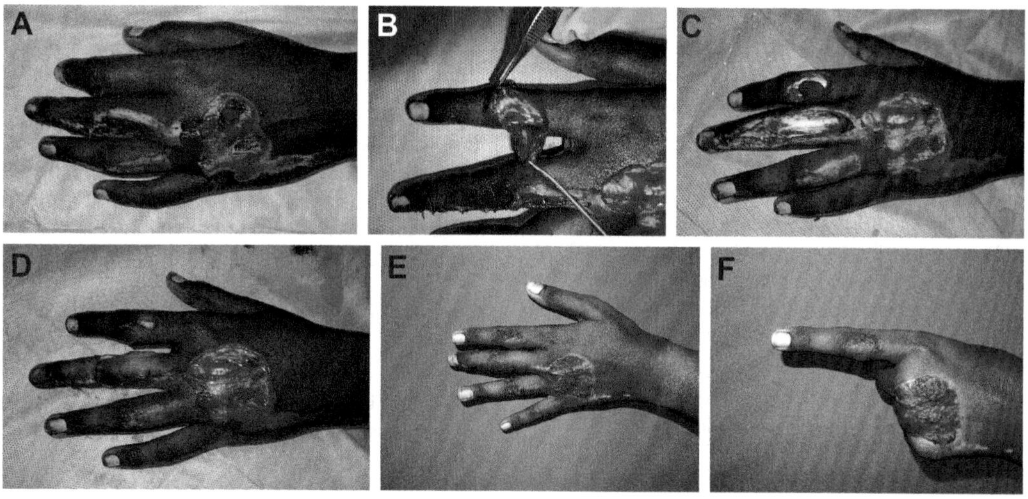

Fig. 10. (*A*) Deep friction injury with skin loss involving index, middle, and ring fingers. (*B*) Proximal interphalangeal joint exposed over index finger along with raised rotational flap. (*C*) Rotational flap raised before transfer for index finger with exposed middle finger extensor tendon. (*D*) Rotational flap inset into defect with transposition flap cover of middle finger. (*E, F*) Final result of rotational and transpositional flap.

It is difficult to raise conventional rotation flaps in the fingers because of a lack of lax skin. Any rotation flap could be considered as having components of both transposition and advancement, and particularly in fingers, it lean toward the transposition end of the spectrum. These flaps are usually used to cover small circular defects over the metacarpophalangeal and interphalangeal joints. When planning a rotation flap, one should keep in mind that a larger flap will be required for defects over the joint to account for the excess skin requirements during flexion (**Fig. 9**). The lateral rotation flaps are marked with the distal margin extending to the midlateral line. Moving more distal on the dorsum of the finger, the size of the flaps reduces. Once the flap rotates (**Fig. 10**), there is a small "dog ear" noted along the proximal edge, which can be trimmed. Differential suturing usually permits linear closure of the donor defect in rotation flaps. However, one should not hesitate to skin graft the donor site, if there is excessive tension. A tie-over dressing is applied over the skin graft and will be removed after 7 days.

Advantages:

- Ideal for circular defects
- Avoids skin grafting of donor area
- Pliability of dorsal skin allows free joint movement
- Good vascularity

Disadvantages:

- Not suitable for larger defects

OUTCOMES

In terms of durability, skin flaps are better than adipofascial flaps. Adipofascial flaps do better when there is a need to fill dead spaces. In designing transposition flaps, one needs to consider limited tissue availability, cylindrical nature of the digit, the need to provide a supple and "tension-free" flap that allows good motion, and the donor defect. Even if the vascularity of the far extent of the flap is partially compromised, it has been observed to heal secondarily. Rotation flaps in the fingers are ideally suited for small circular defects and can be raised along the transfer axis. The results are good, but sometimes a back cut or skin grafting may be needed.

REFERENCES

1. Hynes W. The skin dermis graft as an alternative to the direct or tubed flap. Br J Plast Surg 1954;7:97.
2. Pakiam AJ. The reversed dermis flap. Br J Plast Surg 1978;31(2):131–5.
3. Atasoy E. Reversed cross-finger subcutaneous flap. J Hand Surg 1982;7A:481–3.
4. Thatte RL, Gopalakrishna A, Prasad S. The use of deepithelialised "turn over" flaps in the hand. Br J Plast Surg 1982;35:293–9.
5. Lai C-S, Lin S-D, Yang C-C, et al. The adipofascial turnover flap for complicated dorsal skin defects of the hand and finger. Br J Plast Surg 1991;44:165–9.
6. Yii NW, Elliot D. Bipedicle strap flaps in reconstruction of longitudinal dorsal skin defects of the digits. Plast Reconstr Surg 1999;103:1205–11.

7. Levame JH, Otero C, Berdugo G. Vascularisation arte rielle des te guments de la face dorsale de la main et des doigts. Ann Chir Plast 1967;12:316–24.
8. Smith PJ. A sliding flap to cover dorsal skin defects over the proximal interphalangeal joint. Hand 1982; 14:271–8.
9. Oberlin C, Le Quang G. E tude anatomique de la vascularisation du lambeau en Drapeau. Ann Chir Main 1985;4:169–74.
10. Yousif NJ, Cunningham MW, Sanger JR, et al. The vascular supply to the proximal interphalangeal joint. J Hand Surg 1985;10A:852–61.
11. Valenti P, Masquelet AC, Begué T. Anatomic basis of a dorso-commissural flap from the 2nd, 3rd and 4th intermetacarpal spaces. Surg Radiol Anat 1990;12: 235–9.
12. Strauch B, de Moura W. Arterial system of the fingers. J Hand Surg 1990;15A:148–54.
13. Braga-Silva J. Anatomic basis of dorsal finger skin cover. Tech Hand Up Extrem Surg 2005;9:134–41.
14. Braga-Silva J, Kuyven CR, Fallopa F, et al. An anatomical study of the dorsal cutaneous branches of the digital arteries. J Hand Surg 2002;27B:577–9.
15. Vuppalapati G, Oberlin C, Balakrishnan G. "Distally based dorsal hand flaps": clinical experience, cadaveric studies and an update. Br J Plast Surg 2004;57:653–67.
16. Endo T, Kojima T, Hirase Y. Vascular anatomy of the finger dorsum and a new idea for coverage of the finger pulp defect that restores sensation. J Hand Surg Am 1992;17:927–32.
17. Delia G, Casoli V, Sommario M, et al. Homodigital dorsal adipofascial reverse flap: anatomical study of distal perforators and key points for safe dissection. J Hand Surg Eur Vol 2010;35:454–8.
18. Lai CS, Lin SD, Chou CK, et al. A versatile method for reconstruction of finger defects: reverse digital artery flap. Br J Plast Surg 1992;45:443–53.
19. Voche P, Merle M. The homodigital subcutaneous flap for cover of dorsal finger defects. Br J Plast Surg 1994;47:435–9.
20. Lister G. The theory of the transposition flap and its practical application in the hand. Clin Plast Surg 1981;8:115–27.

VY Advancement, Thenar Flap, and Cross-finger Flaps

Jin Xi Lim, MBBS[a,b,*], Kevin C. Chung, MD, MS[c]

KEYWORDS

• VY advancement flap • Thenar flap • Cross-finger flap • Fingertip amputation • Fingertip defects

KEY POINTS

- Fingertip amputations are common injuries with a myriad of management options.
- The VY advancement flap is classically used to cover distal transverse or volar favorable fingertip amputations.
- Volar unfavorable amputations can be reliably resurfaced by thenar or cross-finger flaps.
- Although these flaps are not innervated, patients can have good sensory recovery, especially younger patients.

INTRODUCTION

Fingertip amputations are one of the most common problems presenting for acute care. VY advancement, thenar flaps, and cross-finger flaps are work-horse flaps that are frequently used to resurface fingertip amputations, although they differ in their indications. These flaps are reliable and simple to perform without the need for neurovascular dissection.

VY ADVANCEMENT FLAPS

Historical Review and Variations

The earliest description of the VY advancement flap was by Dr Ettore Tranquilli-Leali[1] in 1935. A variation of this flap was popularized by Atasoy and colleagues[2] in 1970 that differs in its vascular supply. Other variations include the neurovascular Tranquilli-Leali flap,[3–5] in which the flap design extends proximal to the distal interphalangeal crease and the flap is vascularized by the digital artery proper. The flap design was described for fingertip amputations that were proximal to the midnail level and that required a greater flap advancement for coverage.[3] DeJongh[6] described a variation of advancement flap for fingertip defects in which the flap is designed as a rectangle and a transverse incision is made on the pulp about 6 mm parallel and proximal to the amputation. A crescent flap (**Fig. 1**A) was also described for defects for use in situations in which the conventional VY flap would not be adequate for coverage and to preserve fingertip contour.[7]

An alternative method for advancement was described by Snow,[8] Furlow,[9] and Tezel,[10] in which the distal ends of the triangular flap are brought together to form a cup at the end of the

Disclosure: The authors have no commercial or financial conflicts of interest.

[a] Department of Orthopaedic Surgery, Ng Teng Fong General Hospital, National University Health System, Singapore, Singapore; [b] Department of Hand and Reconstructive Microsurgery, National University Health System, 1E Kent Ridge Road, Level 11, Singapore 119228, Singapore; [c] Section of Plastic Surgery, The University of Michigan Medical School, 1500 East Medical Center Drive, 2130 Taubman Center, SPC 5340, Ann Arbor, MI, USA
* Corresponding author. Department of Orthopaedic Surgery, Ng Teng Fong General Hospital, National University health System, Singapore, Singapore.
E-mail address: jin_xi_lim@nuhs.edu.sg

Hand Clin 36 (2020) 19–32
https://doi.org/10.1016/j.hcl.2019.08.003

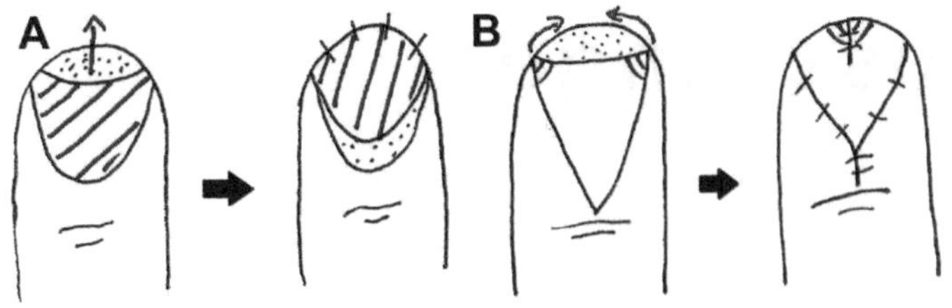

Fig. 1. Alternative flap designs for VY advancement flap. (*A*) Crescent flap. (*B*) VY cup flap.

flap (**Fig. 1**B). This flap provides better coverage with less advancement of the flap and, when the 2 ends of the triangle fold together, the dog ear that results adds bulk and gives better contour to the reconstructed fingertip.

Indications

The volar VY advancement flap can advance about 5 to 7 mm in our experience, and is best used for resurfacing of a fingertip amputation that is either transverse or volar favorable[2] (**Fig. 2**A, B). It is useful in distal fingertip amputations when at least 15 mm of the distal segment of the finger (measured from the distal interphalangeal joint crease) is available for flap advancement. It can also be used to resurface adherent or sensitive scars of the fingertip and hook nail deformity.

Surgical Anatomy

The VY advancement flap is supplied by the terminal branches of the digital artery. In the Tranquilli-Leali flap, a full-thickness incision is made down to the periosteum of the distal phalanx. Therefore, the flap is supplied via the anastomotic connections between the terminal branches of the volar digital arteries and the dorsal arches through the fibro-osseous hiatus branch.[11] The Atasoy variation of this flap is raised by only incising the skin and other fibrous structures, as detailed later, while preserving the terminal branches of the digital artery and nerve.[3,11]

Operative Technique

Our preference is to raise the flap in the manner described by Atasoy and colleagues[2] (**Figs. 2** and **3**):

1. The procedure is done under digital block.
2. Debridement is done. If there is a portion of the distal phalanx protruding beyond the nail bed, the bone is shortened to the level of the nail bed.
3. A triangular flap is designed with the base at the edge of the amputation and its apex at the distal interphalangeal crease (see **Fig. 2**C). The base should be of the same width as the nail bed (see **Fig. 2**D).
4. The skin incision is made first.
5. To get good advancement, the following structures must be divided:
   a. Fibrous tissue at the apex of the flap (see **Fig. 2**E)
   b. Fibrous tissue at both sides of the base of the flap
6. The deep margin of the flap is then separated from the periosteum and the flexor tendon sheath (see **Fig. 2**F).
7. Using a skin hook for traction at the flap base, identify fibrous tissue that is limiting advancement and divide them (see **Fig. 2**G).
8. The flap is then advanced and sutured to the nail bed (see **Fig. 2**H).
9. The proximal portion of the V incision is closed linearly, forming a Y-shaped wound (see **Fig. 2**I–K).

Aesthetic Refinements

Pulp contour

- Linear closure of the donor defect may reduce the circumference of the pulp. To prevent this, the authors recommend either of 2 methods: (1) flap design with a tapered apex (see **Fig. 2**C); (2) allowing the secondary defect to heal by secondary intention.[12]
- The base of the triangular flap should be the width of the nail bed. Raising a flap with narrower base results in problems with the pulp contour, as shown in **Fig. 4**A.

Tip contour and hook nail deformity

The nail bed in a normal digit was shown to be entirely supported by the distal phalanx and none of it rests on soft tissue.[13] Hook nail deformity (**Fig. 4**B) or a beaked nail occurs when there is loss of bony support for the distal nail bed and the excess nail bed curves palmarly at its most distal portion. This deformity is unsightly and may result in difficulties with picking up small objects and nail trimming. To prevent hook nail deformity, nail

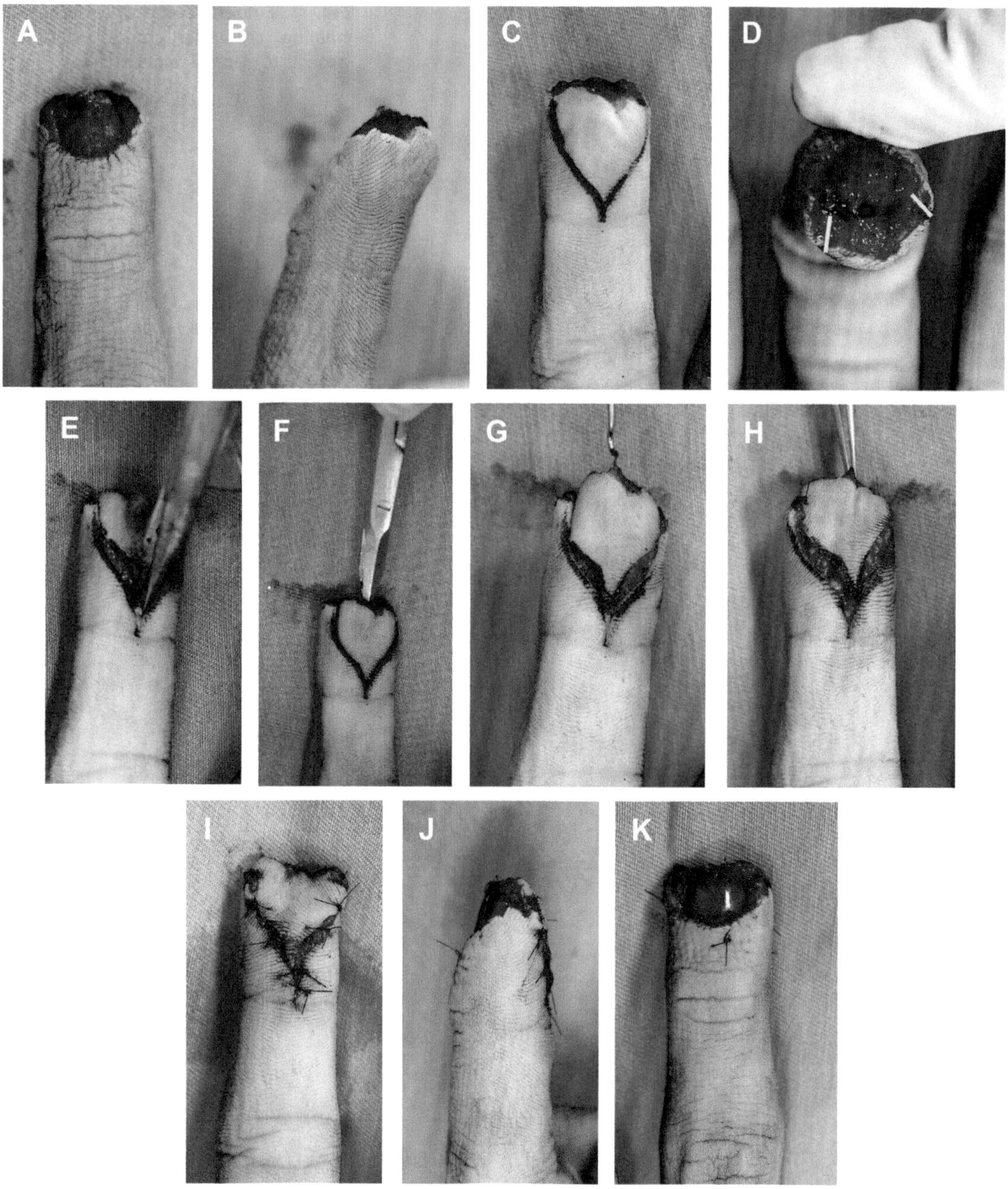

Fig. 2. Steps of raising a VY advancement flap. (*A, B*) Volar neutral fingertip amputation. (*C*) VY flap design. (*D*) Yellow lines represent the lateral limits of the flap, which should be same as the width of the nail bed. (*E*) Division of fibrous tissue at the apex of the flap. (*F*) Separation of the deep margin of the flap from the periosteum and the flexor tendon sheath. (*G*) Using a skin hook for traction at the flap base, fibrous tissue that is limiting advancement is identified and divided. (*H*) The flap is then advanced and sutured to the nail bed. (*I–K*) After flap inset is complete.

beds that extend distal to the tip of the distal phalanx should be excised.

In addition, the authors have advocated the use of Kirschner wires to pin the flap to the distal phalanx instead of direct suture. The flap is advanced to cover the critical area and secured with a pin. The rest of the wound is not closed but left to heal by secondary intention. This technique improves the reach of the flap without excessive risk for flap ischemia. Pulp contour is improved because of the healing by secondary intention.[14]

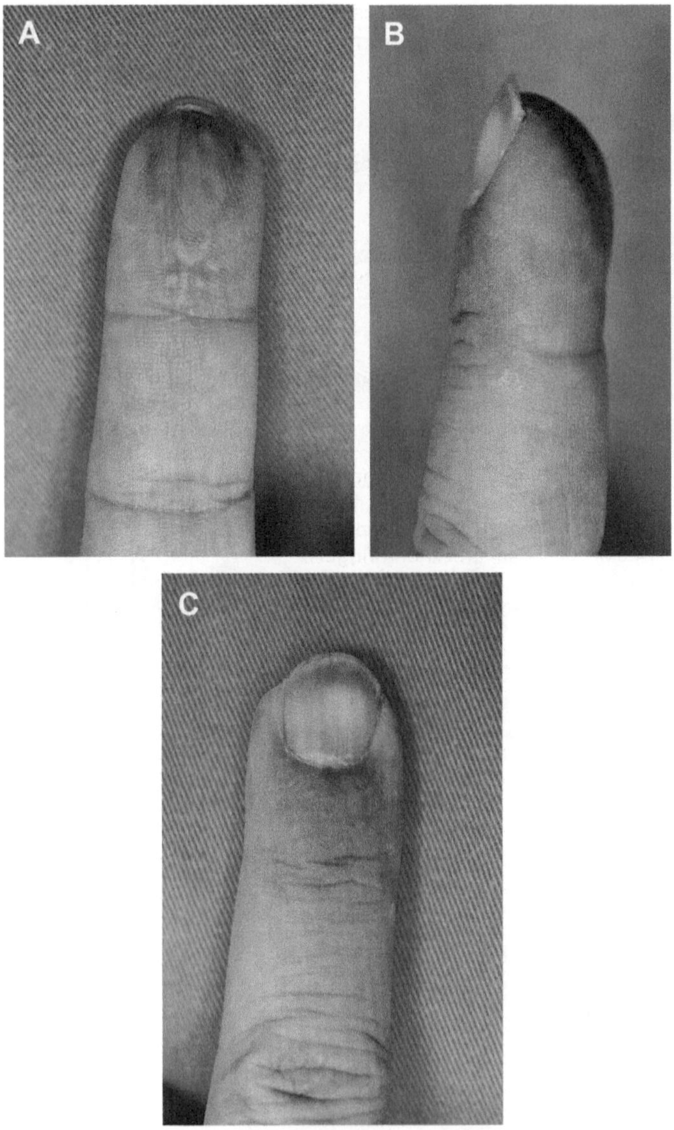

Fig. 3. Fingertip contour after flap healing. (*A*) Volar aspect. (*B*) Lateral aspect. (*C*) Dorsal aspect.

Nail

In a volar favorable fingertip amputation, clinicians might encounter patients with very short remnant nails. To improve the appearance of the fingertip, an eponychial recession can be performed. This technique exposes the portion of the germinal matrix normally hidden by the eponychium, thus making the nail

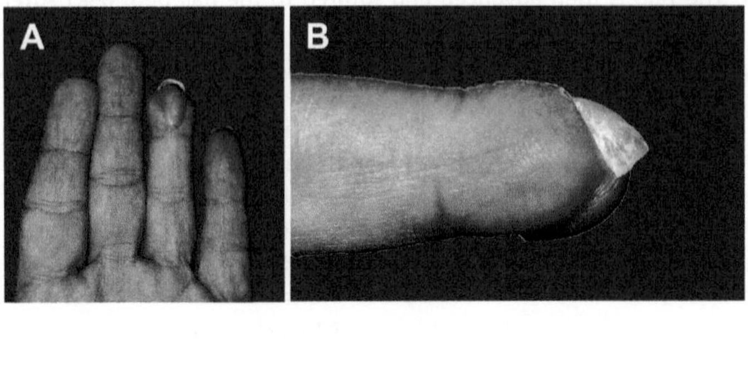

Fig. 4. Complications. (*A*) Result of VY advancement with flap of smaller base. (*B*) Hook nail deformity.

look longer by 2 to 4 mm.[15,16] A crescent-shaped area of skin is excised about 4 to 5 mm proximal to the eponychium. The maximum width of the excised skin is approximately 3 to 4 mm. The wound is then closed linearly, effectively bringing the eponychium to a more proximal position relative to the nail bed (**Fig. 5**).

Outcomes

This flap is simple to perform, reliable, and the donor site can be closed linearly. It also preserves good fingertip sensation with glabrous skin. Atasoy and colleagues[2] reported excellent aesthetic outcomes with normal finger range of motion and normal fingertip sensation in 97% of their patients. In their series of 61 patients, 2 had superficial skin necrosis.[2] In another study of 20 patients with 5.9 years of follow-up, there was an average of 3-mm difference in 2-point discrimination (2 PD) between the injured finger and the contralateral normal fingertip. However, 25% of the fingertips had persistent tenderness and 15% had nail beaking.[17] It would be logical to assume that the

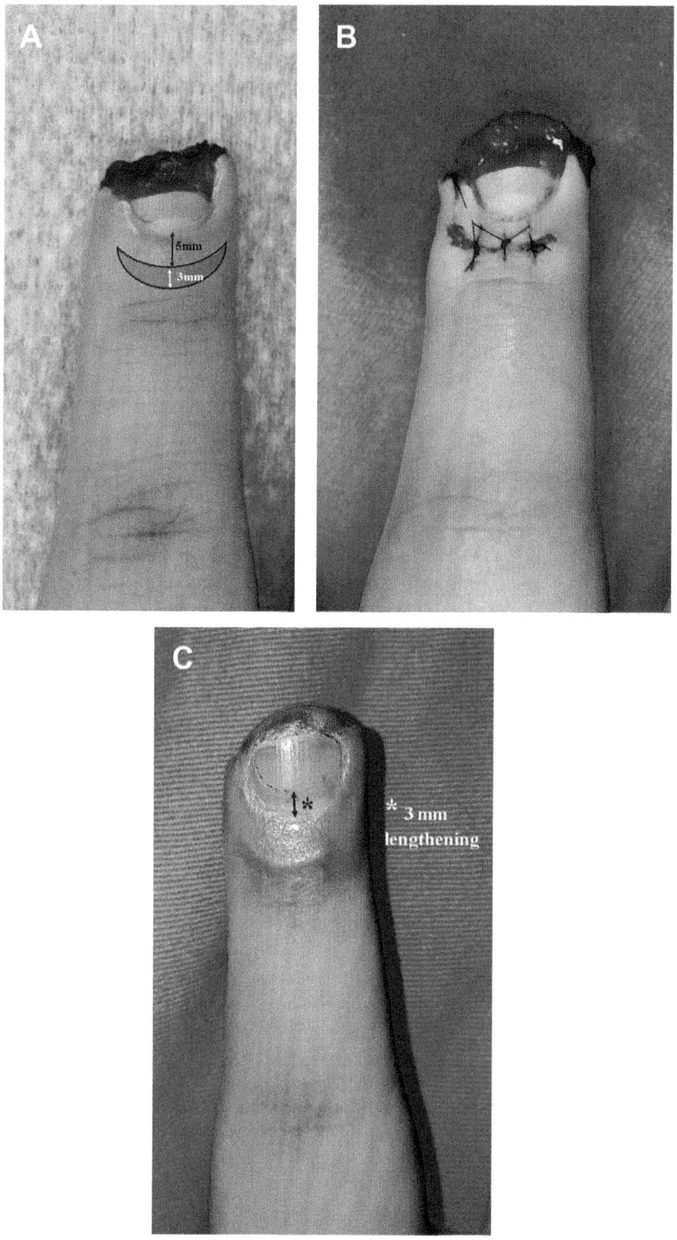

Fig. 5. Eponychial recession. (*A*) Volar favorable fingertip amputation with 3 mm of exposed nail bed. A crescent-shaped area of skin is excised 5 mm proximal to the eponychium with width of 3 mm. (*B*) The resultant wound is then closed directly, effectively recessing the eponychium and exposing 3 mm more of the nail bed. (*C*) Clinical view showing results at 3 months after the procedure.

Tranquilli-Leali technique would give a worse outcome in terms of sensibility because the branches of the digital nerves would be transected during the procedure. However, this has not been proved in the literature.

THENAR FLAPS

Historical Review and Variations

The earliest description of the thenar flap was by Gatewood[18] in 1926. He described an ulnarly based pedicled flap over the thenar eminence that was used to cover a 2 × 2.5-cm defect over the index fingertip. The donor defect was closed linearly and the flap was divided at 12 days after the initial surgery. Since then, flaps that are distally based,[19] proximally based,[20] and H shaped[21] have been described. Investigators have also used double thenar flaps for coverage of multiple fingertip defects and have shown that the results are comparable with those of doing only a single thenar flap.[22] Thenar perforator flaps have also been described. Akita and colleagues[23] stated that the inclusion of a perforator allowed a longer and larger flap to be raised, which, in turn, allowed the finger joints to be in lesser degrees of flexion and potentially less stiffness in the injured digit.

Indications

The thenar flap can be used to cover volar unfavorable fingertip amputations and more extensive pulp losses of the involving the index, middle, and ring finger. It can also be used to cover defects of the nail bed.

Surgical Anatomy

The thenar flap is a random pattern flap and does not need any specific vascular dissection. However, knowledge of detailed vascular anatomy and sensory innervation allows surgeons to raise perforator and free flaps from this area.

The vascular anatomy of the thenar eminence was shown by Omokawa and colleagues[24] in a cadaveric study. The skin over the thenar eminence was supplied by the superficial palmar branch of the radial artery. The skin territory supplied by this vessel was 5.1 × 3.4 cm on average. The average diameter of the artery at its origin was about 1.4 mm with a pedicle length of 2 cm. The superficial palmar branch also had connections to other arteries in the palm in 63% of the specimens. The thenar eminence is drained via one of 3 routes: venae comitantes of the superficial palmar branch of the radial artery, superficial veins from the dorsal border of the thenar eminence, and superficial palmar veins that drain into the superficial forearm median vein. Sensory innervation of the thenar eminence is mainly supplied by the palmar cutaneous branch of the median nerve. There are also contributions from the lateral antebrachial cutaneous nerve and superficial radial nerve in varying degrees.

Operative Technique

1. The procedure can be done under a wrist block.
2. After thorough debridement of the injured fingertip, the digit is flexed so that the defect leaves an imprint on the thenar eminence (**Figs. 6** and **7**A).
3. The authors typically raise this flap as a distally based flap. The distal end of a proximally based flap is inset into the nail bed, whereas the distal end of a distally based flap is inset into the pulp. We prefer a distally based flap because we think that the distally based flap allows inset over a larger surface area. Care must be taken to avoid injuring the radial digital nerve of the thumb. Avoid raising a flap close to first web to prevent web space contractures. The secondary defect is closed linearly (**Fig. 7**B).
4. Flap inset (**Fig. 7**C) is done over the proximal and lateral aspects of the finger defect and dressings applied. It is important to ensure that the flap does not get kinked while in the dressings.

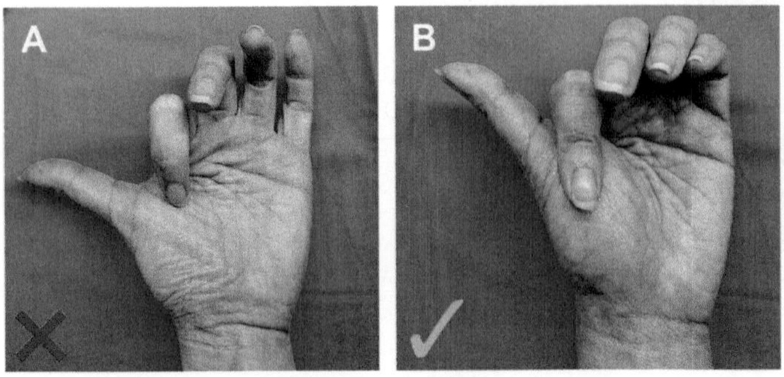

Fig. 6. Siting of donor site. (*A*) Incorrect location of thenar flap. This is too near to the first web space and the thumb base and poses danger to the neurovascular bundle of the thumb. (*B*) The correct location of the flap should be more proximal, over the thenar area. This location prevents scar contractures of the thumb and first web space.

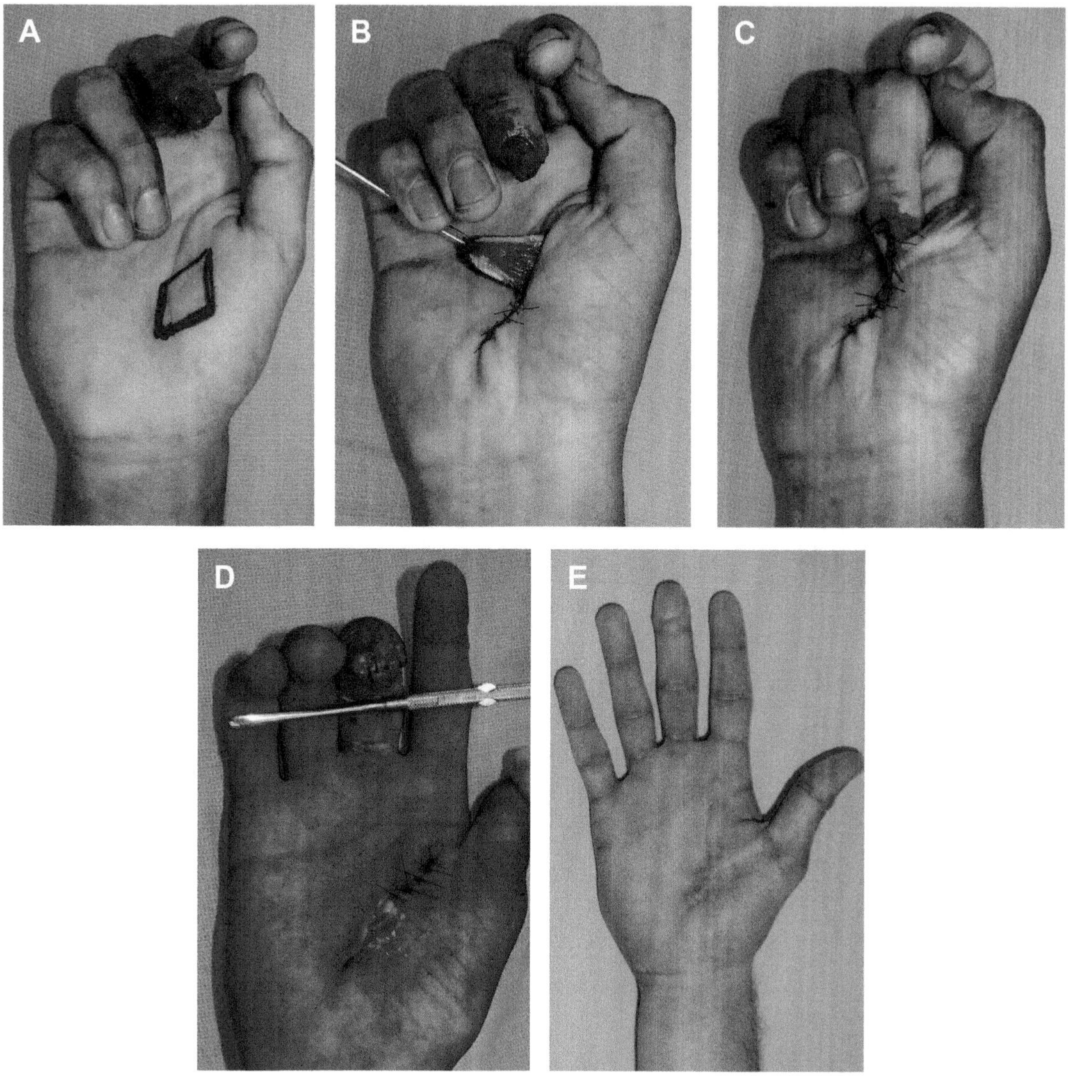

Fig. 7. Thenar flap. (*A*) Flap design: rhomboid-shaped flap is outlined at the proximal thenar eminence. (*B*) Flap is raised with linear closure of donor site. (*C*) Flap inset. (*D*) Flap division. (*E*) Results at 4 months after surgery.

5. Flap division is performed 2 to 3 weeks later (**Fig. 7**D, E).

Aesthetic Refinements

Primary closure of the secondary defect can be made easier by designing either a rhomboid or H-shaped flap, instead of a rectangular flap design. As far as possible, the flap donor site should be more proximal on the thenar eminence to prevent scar contractures of the thumb or the first web space (see **Fig. 6**).

Outcomes

A major advantage of this flap is the presence of good tissue matching with glabrous skin and easy flap dissection. The secondary defect has a healthy muscle bed and is easily closed linearly or using a skin graft. The scarring at the donor site is usually inconspicuous. Disadvantages includes stiffness of the digit, injury to digital nerve to the thumb, and donor site scar contracture and sensitivity. In general, all reported series of the thenar flap have good aesthetic outcomes, good sensory recovery, with absent to minimal finger stiffness and donor site problems. Raising the flap distally, proximally, or laterally did not seem to affect outcomes (**Table 1**).

CROSS-FINGER FLAPS

Historical Review

The cross-finger flap is a 2-staged procedure first published by Gurdin and Pangman[31] in 1950 but

Table 1
Results of thenar flaps

Author, Year	N	Age (y)	Division (d)	Follow-up (y)	Sensation (mm)	ROM	Complications at Donor Site	Design
Miller,[25] 1974	32	3–67	14 (10–21)	4	Static 2 PD 3 patients: 4 5 patients: 4–5 2 patients: 5–6 8 patients: nil (only done in 18 patients)	1% of patients with DIPJ stiffness. No PIPJ stiffness noted	NR	Proximally based
Melone et al,[26] 1982	150	35 (2–73)	10–14	>1	Static 2 PD: 7	4% of patients with stiffness (none was a direct result of the procedure)	1% of patients with sensitive scar	Proximally based
Dellon,[19] 1983	5	22 (18–31)	21	3	Static 2 PD: 6 (4–10) Moving 2 PD: 3 (3–4)	No residual finger stiffness	Nil complications	Distally based
Fitoussi et al,[27] 2004	12	4 (2–11)	22 (18–25)	2 (1–3)	Static 2 PD 5 (4–9)	No joint contractures	No flap necrosis, no donor site morbidity	Distally based
Okazaki et al,[28] 2005	8	40 (11–57)	14 (12–17)	1	Moving 2 PD: <6	No PIPJ contracture	No scar contracture	Distally based
Rinker,[29] 2006	17	21 (3–48)	13 (10–15)	NR	Static 2 PD 6 (3–10)	Not significantly reduced compared with contralateral side	17% cold intolerance	Radially based
Barr et al,[30] 2014	16	11 (1–18)	16 (12–24)	6.8 mo (4.1–9.6 mo)	Static 2 PD 7 (6–10)[a]	Average total active motion 248° (235°–260°)	No flap necrosis, no donor site morbidity	Proximally based

Abbreviations: NR, not reported; PD, point discrimination; PIPJ, proximal interphalangeal joint; ROM, range of motion.
[a] For patients who were cooperative with sensory testing.
Data from Refs.[16,25–30]

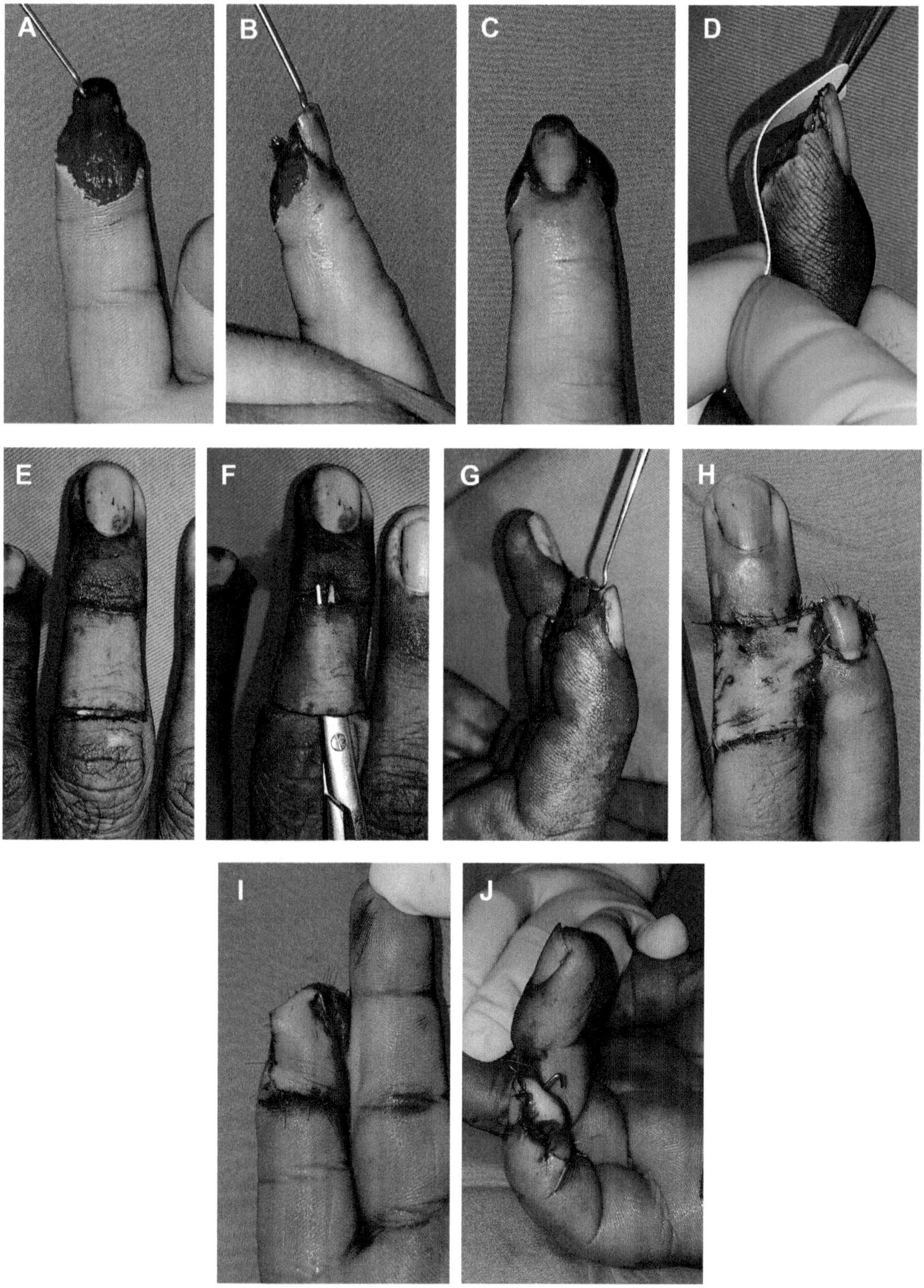

Fig. 8. Cross-finger flap. (*A–C*) Volar unfavorable fingertip defect. (*D*) Excess skin is needed to recreate the pulp contour. (*E*) The proximal and distal extent of the flap is incised first and dissection is carried down to the paratenon of the extensor tendon. (*F*) The flap is then separated from the paratenon with blunt dissection. (*G*) To get good fingertip contour, anchor the sides of the flap at the lateral aspect of the distal-most region of the defect first and leave about 5 mm of excess flap hanging out distally. After the proximal part of the flap inset is done, the tip is turned down and then sutured to the sterile matrix. (*H*) A full-thickness skin graft is then harvested and used to cover the flap donor defect and the exposed skin bridge. (*I, J*) Flap inset is complete.

was used by Cronin[32] as an original procedure since 1945. The flap is taken from the dorsum of an adjacent digit, usually at the level of the middle phalanx, and is used to resurface a volar unfavorable pulp amputation. This flap does not require the patient to place the arm in an awkward position, and is also easier to perform and less time consuming than raising an island flap.

The innervated cross-finger flap was first published by Adamson and colleagues[33] in 1967. The flap was harvested from the index finger along with branches of the superficial radial nerve to cover the thumb pulp. This technique was described with the aim of providing sensation to the thumb. A dual-innervated flap was also described.[34] The dual innervation originates from branches of the superficial radial nerve as well as the dorsal branch of the digital nerve proper. The dorsal branch of the proper radial digital nerve is cut and then neurotized to the thumb ulnar digital nerve to provide a dual source of innervation.

Indications

The cross-finger flap is reliable and has the ability to cover extensive loss of the pulp of the fingers and the thumb (**Fig. 8**A–C). It can also cover defects at any level of the digit, unlike the thenar flap, which can only resurface defects at the fingertip. It is limited only by the amount of available skin from the donor digit; the width is limited by the midlateral line of the digit, and the maximum length extends from the level of the distal interphalangeal joint to the level of the palmodigital crease.

Surgical Anatomy

The cross-finger flap was initially raised as a random pattern flap. Investigators advised respecting the flap length/width ratio during flap harvest to ensure flap viability. However, consistent dorsal branches of the digital artery were described in 1990 by Strauch and Moura.[35] The anatomy of the dorsal branches of the digital artery was further detailed by Braga-silva and colleagues,[36] who described 4 constant dorsal branches arising at predictable distances from the proximal interphalangeal joint. The skin from the dorsum of the finger can be harvested as an island flap because of the presence of these branches.

Sensory innervation of the dorsum of a finger has 2 main contributions: 1 from the dorsal branches of the digital nerve proper, the second from branches of either the superficial radial nerve or dorsal branch of ulnar nerve.

Operative Technique

1. The procedure can be done under a digital block or wrist block (**Fig. 8**).
2. After debridement of the injured fingertip, the defect size is measured.
3. For a pulp defect, the flap is designed on the dorsum of the middle phalanx of an adjacent digit. Choice of donor digit usually respects the natural finger cascade after flap inset. Keep in mind that some excess tissue has to be taken to get good pulp contour (see **Fig. 8**D).
4. The proximal and distal extent of the flap is incised first and dissection is carried down to the paratenon of the extensor tendon (see **Fig. 8**E). The flap is then separated from the paratenon with blunt dissection (see **Fig. 8**F). A rectangular flap is harvested, leaving the edge of the flap closest to the recipient finger intact. It is important to ensure the paratenon

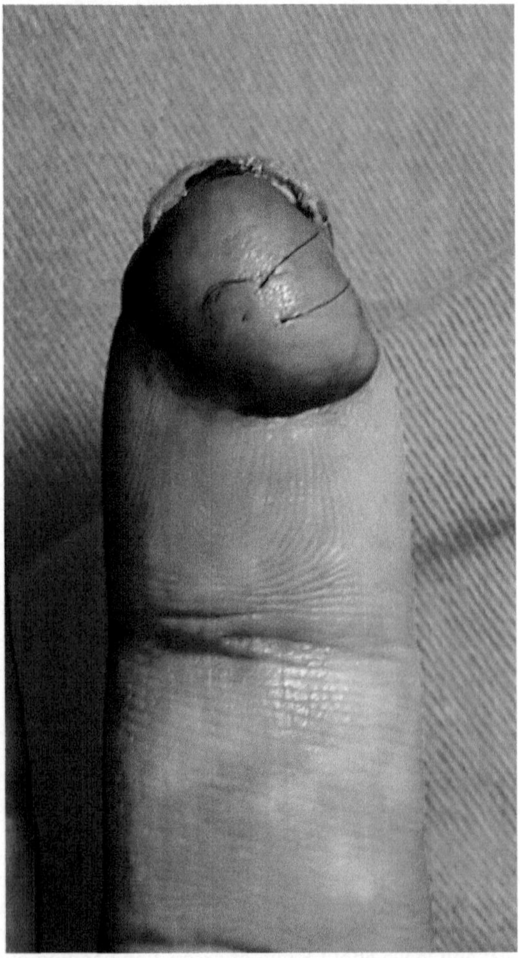

Fig. 9. If flap is too small, the circular scar will contract with time and result in a bulbous flap.

Table 2
Results of cross-finger flaps

Author, Year	N	Age (y)	Division (d)	Follow-up (y)	Sensation	Range of Motion in Donor Finger	Complication	Design
Bralliar & Horner,[39] 1969	14	17–59	21	2 (0.2–5)	86% 2 PD 9 mm (2–19) 14% 2 PD not measurable	NR	15% had hypersensitivity of pulp preventing use of digit	Single-innervated cross-finger flap
Kleinert et al,[38] 1974	56	1–67	12–14	NR	59% had 2 PD of <6 mm	12.5% with limitation in motion	NR	Standard cross-finger flap
Nicolai & Hentenaar,[37] 1981	51	30 (1–63)	21.6 (15–28)	NR	35 patients: ≤6 mm difference compared with uninjured finger	NR	59% with cold sensitivity	Standard cross-finger flap
Nishikawa & Smith,[40] 1992	28	NR	NR	2 (1–4)	Average of 70% subjective recovery	60% had subjective stiffness but no measurable loss	53% with cold sensitivity	Standard cross-finger flap
Paterson et al,[41] 2000	16	41 (6–59)	12–17	4 (1–9)	NR	50% with limitation in motion	62.5% cold sensitivity (at donor site)	Standard cross-finger flap
Koch et al,[42] 2005	23	30 (2–59)	NR	7 (2–18)	NR	Total ROM Donor: 156° (20°–235°) Control: 174° (95°–270°)	30.4% cold sensitivity (at donor site)	Standard cross-finger flap
Rabarin et al,[43] 2016	22	59 (27–82)	15	20 (17—23)	No subjective difference in sensation 2 PD: 9 patients, no difference 5 patients, 2-mm difference 2 patients, 4-mm difference	No interphalangeal joint flexion stiffness	No flap necrosis, infection or wound dehiscence 31.8% with cold sensitivity	Standard cross-finger flap

Data from Refs.[4,37–39,41–43]

of the extensor tendon is left intact to have good take of the skin graft.

5. Flap inset is then performed. To get good fingertip contour, one suggestion is to anchor the sides of the flap at the lateral aspect of the distal defect first and to leave about 5 mm of excess flap hanging out distally (see **Fig. 8**G). After the proximal part of the flap inset is done, the tip is turned down and then sutured to the sterile matrix.
6. A full-thickness skin graft is then harvested and used to cover the secondary defect and the exposed skin bridge (see **Fig. 8**H). A tie-over dressing is then placed over the skin graft recipient site.
7. Dressings are then applied and there is no need for any immobilization.

The second stage is usually done 2 to 3 weeks later. It is imperative to ensure good dermal healing at the recipient site before flap division.

1. The procedure is done under a wrist block.
2. After cleaning the operative site, the base of the flap is divided, ensuring adequate skin for coverage of the defect.
3. The cut edge of the flap is shaped, defatted to ensure good contour, and closed primarily.
4. The cut edge of the flap at the donor site is also trimmed and closed primarily.
5. Dressings are placed and early range-of-motion exercises are started.

Aesthetic Refinements

Typically flaps are designed to match the defect. However, in the cross-finger flap, the defect must be matched to the flap. In a smaller or irregularly sized defect, the defect should be enlarged to match the rectangular shape of the cross-finger flap. This process often requires excision of some normal skin. In addition, covering a circular defect in the pulp with a cross-finger flap often results in an unsightly bulbous flap caused by circular scar contracture (**Fig. 9**). Enlarging the defect also allows a flap with a larger base to be raised. If the flap donor site is a dense hair-bearing area, a cross-finger flap might not be a suitable choice for the patient because hair will then grow on the pulp after transfer of the tissue.

Note that hair will also continue to grow on full-thickness skin grafts and will be similar to the density at the donor site. Therefore, choice of skin graft donor site is important to ensure that the appearance of the donor site will be more aesthetically pleasing. Common areas for donor sites include the distal wrist crease, cubital fossa, and the proximal medial forearm. The authors do not harvest skin graft from the distal wrist crease because the scar resembles the scar of a self-inflicted wound and may be stigmatizing to some patients.

Outcomes

The main criticism of the cross-finger flap is that it is a 2-staged procedure, uses an uninjured digit, and may result in stiffness of the donor finger. In addition, it does not provide glabrous skin for coverage. Although the flap is not an innervated flap, it has been shown that this flap can achieve good sensory recovery and good results with younger patients.[37,38] In addition, a handful of studies reported having no reduced range of motion of the donor digit (**Table 2**).

In the 2 cases reported by Hastings[34] on the use of a dual-innervated cross-finger flap to resurface the thumb pulp, 1 patient obtained a 2 PD of 5 mm at 1.5 years and the other achieved this at 7 months.

SUMMARY

The VY advancement, thenar, and cross-finger flaps are all reliable and easy to raise. All 3 flaps gave consistently good results in terms of sensitivity. Comparing thenar and cross-finger flaps, the thenar flap gives better return of sensibility because of the higher density of nerve endings in the palmar skin, whereas the cross-finger flap is usually harvested from the dorsum of a digit. Flap division can be safely done at 2 to 3 weeks with very few reports of flap necrosis. It is postulated that earlier flap division may reduce the degree of stiffness in the donor and recipient digit. The VY advancement flap is only indicated in distal transverse or volar favorable fingertip amputations. The thenar and cross-finger flaps can cover a bigger defect, but both require a 2-stage procedure. Other alternatives that can be considered for similar-sized defects include neurovascular island flaps, reverse vascular island flaps, heterodigital neurovascular island flaps, and free flaps. However, these flaps require microvascular dissection and a higher level of expertise.

REFERENCES

1. Tranquilli-Leali E. Ricostruzione dell'apice delle falangi ungueali mediante autoplastica volare peduncolata per scorrimento. Infort Traumatol Lav 1935; 1:186–93.
2. Atasoy E, Ioakimidis E, Kasdan ML, et al. Reconstruction of the amputated finger tip with a triangular

volar flap. A new surgical procedure. J Bone Joint Surg Am 1970;52:921–6.
3. Elliot D, Moiemen NS, Jigjinni VS. The neurovascular Tranquilli-Leali flap. J Hand Surg Br 1995;20(6): 815–23.
4. O'connor D, Samuel AW. Finger flaps: using the modified neurovascular Tranquilli-Leali flap. Injury 1998;29(7):564–6.
5. Loréa P, Chahidi N, Marchesi S, et al. Reconstruction of fingertip defects with the neurovascular tranquilli-leali flap. J Hand Surg Br 2006;31(3): 280–4.
6. DeJongh E. A simple plastic procedure of the fingers for conserving bony tissue and forming a soft tissue pad. Am J Surg 1942;57(2): 346–7.
7. Chung SR, Foo TL. Crescent flap for fingertip reconstruction. Hand Surg 2014;19(3):459–61.
8. Snow JW. The use of a volar flap for repair of fingertip amputations: a preliminary report. Comment. Plast Reconstr Surg 1973;52(3):299.
9. Furlow LT. V-Y "Cup" flap for volar oblique amputation of fingers. J Hand Surg Br 1984;9(3): 253–6.
10. Tezel E, Numanoğlu A. A new swing of the atasoy volar V-Y flap. Ann Plast Surg 2001;47(4): 470–1.
11. Gharb BB, Rampazzo A, Armijo BS, et al. Tranquilli-Leali or Atasoy flap: an anatomical cadaveric study. J Plast Reconstr Aesthet Surg 2010;63(4): 681–5.
12. Thoma A, Vartija LK. Making the V-Y advancement flap safer in fingertip amputations. Can J Plast Surg 2010;18(4):e47–9.
13. Kumar VP, Satku K. Treatment and prevention of "hook nail" deformity with anatomic correlation. J Hand Surg Am 1993;18(4):617–20.
14. Foo TL, Wan KH, Chew WY. Safe and easy method to preserve fingertip contour in VY-plasty. Tech Hand Up Extrem Surg 2012; 16(2):95–7.
15. Xing S, Shen Z, Jia W, et al. Aesthetic and functional results from nailfold recession following fingertip amputations. J Hand Surg Am 2015; 40(1):1–7.
16. Adani R, Marcoccio I, Tarallo L. Nail lengthening and fingertip amputations. Plast Reconstr Surg 2003; 112(5):1287–94.
17. Tupper J, Miller G. Sensitivity following volar V-Y plasty for fingertip amputations. J Hand Surg Br 1985;10(2):183–4.
18. Gatewood A. Plastic repair of finger defects without hospitalisation. JAMA 1926;87(18):1479.
19. Dellon AL. The proximal inset thenar flap for fingertip reconstruction. Plast Reconstr Surg 1983;72(5): 698–704.
20. Flatt AE. The thenar flap. J Bone Joint Surg Br 1957; 39-B(1):80–5.
21. Smith RJ, Albin R. Thenar "H-flap" for fingertip injuries. J Trauma 1976;16(10):778–81.
22. Kwon YJ, Ahn BM, Lee JS, et al. Reconstruction of two fingertip amputations using a double thenar flap and comparison of outcomes of surgery using a single thenar flap. Injury 2017; 48(2):481–5.
23. Akita S, Kuroki T, Yoshimoto S, et al. Reconstruction of a fingertip with a thenar perforator island flap. J Plast Surg Hand Surg 2011;45(6): 294–9.
24. Omokawa S, Ryu J, Tang JB, et al. Vascular and neural anatomy of the thenar area of the hand: its surgical applications. Plast Reconstr Surg 1997;99: 116–21.
25. Miller AJ. Single finger tip injuries treated by thenar flap. Hand 1974;6(3):311–4.
26. Melone CP, Beasley RW, Carstens JH. The thenar flap–An analysis of its use in 150 cases. J Hand Surg Am 1982;7(3):291–7.
27. Fitoussi F, Ghorbani A, Jehanno P, et al. Thenar flap for severe finger tip injuries in children. J Hand Surg Br 2004;29(2):108–12.
28. Okazaki M, Hasegawa H, Kano M, et al. A different method of fingertip reconstruction with the thenar flap. Plast Reconstr Surg 2005;115(3):885–8.
29. Rinker B. Fingertip reconstruction with the laterally based thenar flap: indications and long-term functional results. Hand (N Y) 2006;1(1):2–8.
30. Barr JS, Chu MW, Thanik V, et al. Pediatric thenar flaps: a modified design, case series and review of the literature. J Pediatr Surg 2014;49(9):1433–8.
31. Gurdin M, Pangman WJ. The repair of surface defects of fingers by transdigital flaps. Plast Reconstr Surg 1950;5:308–71.
32. Cronin TD. The cross finger flap, a new method of repair. Am Surg 1951;17:419–25.
33. Adamson JE, Horton CE, Crawford HH. Sensory rehabilitation of the injured thumb. Plast Reconstr Surg 1967;40(1):53–7.
34. Hastings H. Dual innervated index to thumb cross finger or island flap reconstruction. Microsurgery 1987;8(3):168–72.
35. Strauch B, Moura W. Arterial system of the fingers. J Hand Surg Am 1990;1:148–54.
36. Braga-silva J, Kuyven CR, Fallopa F, et al. An anatomical study of the dorsal cutaneous branches of the digital arteries. J Hand Surg Br 2002;27(6): 577–9.
37. Nicolai JP, Hentenaar G. Sensation in cross-finger flaps. Hand 1981;13(1):12–6.
38. Kleinert HE, McAlister CG, MacDonald CJ, et al. A critical evaluation of crossfinger flaps. J Trauma 1974;14(9):756–63.

39. Bralliar F, Horner RL. Sensory cross-finger pedicle graft. J Bone Joint Surg Am 1969;51(7):1264–8.
40. Nishikawa H, Smith PJ. The recovery of sensation and function after cross-finger flaps for fingertip injury. J Hand Surg Br 1992;17(1):102–7.
41. Paterson P, Titley OG, Nancarrow JD. Donor finger morbidity in cross-finger flaps. Injury 2000;31(4):215–8.
42. Koch H, Kielnhofer A, Hubmer M, et al. Donor site morbidity in cross-finger flaps. Br J Plast Surg 2005;58(8):1131–5.
43. Rabarin F, Saint cast Y, Jeudy J, et al. Cross-finger flap for reconstruction of fingertip amputations: long-term results. Orthop Traumatol Surg Res 2016;102(4 Suppl):S225–8.

Antegrade Flow Digital Artery Flaps

Poi Hoon Tay, MBChB, David M.K. Tan, MBBS, MMed (Surgery)*

KEYWORDS

- Neurovascular island flaps • Digital artery flaps • Heterodigital island flaps
- Digital island flow-through flaps

KEY POINTS

- Antegrade flow digital artery flaps offer a versatile single-stage reconstruction with the ability to resurface critical defects in homodigital or heterodigital fashion and the palm or dorsum of the hand.
- Variations include the neurovascular island flap for a sensate reconstruction, fasciocutaneous digital artery flaps for larger defects, and as a flow-through flap for concomitant soft tissue coverage and revascularization.
- Disadvantages of this flap include the need to sacrifice a digital artery, the risk of venous congestion, interphalangeal joint contracture, cold intolerance, and incomplete sensory switching when used as a heterodigital transfer.

INTRODUCTION

Soft tissue loss in the hand and its digits can arise from various causes and the variable size and location of critical defects may sometimes preclude the use of simpler strategies, such as skin grafts, local advancement, and rotational or transposition flaps. An islanded flap based on the digital artery offers the following advantages:

1. A constant and robust vascular supply via a proper digital artery with venous drainage via accompanying venae commitantes and perivascular venules.
2. The digital artery and its rich network of branching vessels to the glabrous and dorsal skin of the digit in the proximal and middle phalanx allow the harvest of small to large flaps composed of palmar skin, dorsal skin, or both along with fascial extensions.
3. Islanding a flap on the digital artery allows its transfer to varying locations on the same digit, an adjacent or distant digit, or on some distant part of the hand.
4. The accompanying digital nerve is easily elevated together with the artery and permits restoration of sensation.
5. The distal end of the digital artery may be used to revascularize another digit with a critical arterial injury and concomitant soft tissue defect.

HISTORICAL REVIEW

The concept of elevating an islanded flap based on an antegrade flow digital arterial supply is credited to Moberg[1] and Littler,[2] who described its use as a neurovascular pedicle flap for resurfacing concomitant soft tissue defects and restoring sensation in the thumb, rendered anesthetic by injury.

In 1961, Tubiana and Duparc[3] described the use of the antegrade flow heterodigital neurovascular island flap, outlining the guiding principles in selecting donor tissue, technique of flap elevation, and role of such flaps as part of osteoplastic thumb reconstructions. They also observed that sensory cortical remapping did not occur in 4 of

Disclosure: None.
Department of Hand and Reconstructive Microsurgery, National University Hospital, Level 11, National University Health System Tower Block, 1E Kent Ridge Road, Singapore 119228, Singapore
* Corresponding author.
E-mail address: david_mk_tan@nuhs.edu.sg

Hand Clin 36 (2020) 33–46
https://doi.org/10.1016/j.hcl.2019.08.004

hand.theclinics.com

10 recipient digits. In 1960, Peacock[4] gave the first description of a variation of the island flap based solely on the antegrade flow digital vessel leaving its accompanying digital nerve in situ for the purpose of resurfacing tissue loss in the digits or the palm.

Not long after, Moberg[5] gave the first description of a bipedicled advancement flap as a simple method of sensory reconstruction for an insensate thumb tip by elevating a volar skin flap with its neurovascular elements after having excised the insensate distal skin. O'Brien[6] described its use in both the thumb and finger, only in his case, the volar skin flap was incised to allow more distal advancement, making this a true islanded bipedicled antegrade flow digital artery flap. O'Brien also gave attention to the detail of preserving the dorsal branches of the digital artery to preserve the vascularity of the dorsum of the digit.

Subsequently, various modifications of the neurovascular island flap were described in the literature. Joshi[7] and Pho[8] described a homodigital dorsolateral neurovascular island flap. Harvesting the donor flap from the same digit as the injured finger gradually became popular because this technique avoided donor morbidity in another uninjured digit. Venkataswami and Subramaniam[9] described an oblique triangular advancement flap based on the glabrous skin of the same digit adjacent to the defect for oblique amputations of fingertips in 1980. Later in 1989, Foucher and coworkers[10] described a similar flap based on a single neurovascular pedicle with the exception that the neurovascular bundle was freed and mobilized until the base of the digit to allow more distal advancement. Foucher also proposed the use of the flap as an "exchange flap" elevating the flap from the blind side of the digit to resurface the contact side.

Rose[11] in 1983 expounded further on Peacock's idea and gave detailed technical descriptions and demonstrated six cases in which an islanded flap based solely on the antegrade flow digital artery leaving its accompanying nerve in situ was performed. He termed this the arterialized island pedicle flap and emphasized that careful preservation of the venules accompanying the digital artery through microsurgical dissection technique would prevent venous congestion.

In 1996, Tsai and Yuen[12] described a variation of existing homodigital neurovascular island flaps for resurfacing fingertip loss by harvesting a flap composed of volar, lateral, and dorsal skin proximal to the distal interphalangeal joint based on a single neurovascular bundle and obliquely advancing it to resurface the fingertip. Lim[13] described a similar flap a decade later; however, this differed in that the dorsal skin segment and volar skin segmented is elevated off the whole of the middle phalanx. He and his coauthors purported this allowed better advancement because it facilitated more proximal neurovascular bundle dissection and it had better earlier sensibility because a larger flap incorporated more sensory nerve endings.

Further modifications to the technique of the arterialized island pedicle flap were described by Teoh and coworkers[14] in which a distinct venous supply was included by means of either dissection of an accompanying dorsal vein and transferring it together with the skin island or dividing that accompanying vein and reanastomosing it to a vein adjacent to the recipient bed.[15]

INDICATION/CONTRAINDICATIONS

The antegrade flow digital artery flap is a good and versatile single-stage reconstructive option for resurfacing critical soft tissue defects in the digits and the hand with the option of being a sensate reconstruction by inclusion of the digital nerve accompanying the artery. When defects are situated on a digit other than the one from which the flap is being elevated, consideration should be given for simpler local reconstructive options if they exist because more dissection is required in distant or heterodigital transfers. The breadth of indications is briefly touched on in the Author's preference section.

This flap should be avoided in patients with peripheral vascular disease and vasospastic condition, such as Raynaud disease. Diabetes and tobacco use is not an absolute contraindication for this procedure. Patients with previous injury to the same digit should be carefully evaluated by a digital Allen test before surgery or objectively through imaging to ascertain patency of both digital arteries. Finger stiffness or arthritis is a relative contraindication for this flap.

SURGICAL ANATOMY

A description of the relevant surgical anatomy has been comprehensively covered elsewhere in this issue in the article on vascular anatomy of the hand in relation to flaps. There are, however, several points worth emphasizing:

1. The retrotendinous communicating branches between the digital arteries must be ligated and divided to adequately mobilize the digital island flap.

2. Grayson and Cleland ligaments must be divided to access the digital neurovascular bundle and permit mobilization.
3. The branch of the common digital artery away from the flap must be ligated and divided to allow elevation of the pedicle to the superficial arch.
4. The common digital nerve must be dissected from its branching point distally to proximally to allow adequate pedicle mobilization in a heterodigital neurovascular island flap. This is done by intraneural fasicular dissection using microsurgical technique.

CATEGORIES OF ANTEGRADE FLOW DIGITAL ARTERY FLAPS

These are divided broadly into three categories: (1) homodigital unipedicled island flaps, (2) heterodigital island flaps, and (3) homodigital bipedicled island flaps. The flaps most commonly performed in each category are described including important variations or modifications and some of the outcomes and complications.

Homodigital Unipedicled Island Flaps

Homodigital neurovascular island flap

This flap is harvested from the injured finger itself limiting the morbidity to the same digit. In our practice, we use Foucher's[10] technique. This flap is best indicated for partial fingertip loss, especially oblique fingertip amputations (**Fig. 1**) and volar fingertip skin loss. The vascular pedicle is either the radial or ulnar digital artery. It provides a sensate fingertip reconstruction that is composed of well-padded glabrous skin.

Operative technique Small to modest sized defects are appropriate for resurfacing with this flap and flap advancement of up to 1.5 cm and flap widths up to 1 cm are safely performed (**Fig. 2**). The choice of which digital neurovascular bundle to base the flap on is determined by the location and the size of the defect. We generally prefer flap elevation on the same side as the defect in oblique fingertip wounds and in transverse fingertip loss, on the side where the digital artery is dominant (ulnar in the index and radial in the small finger).

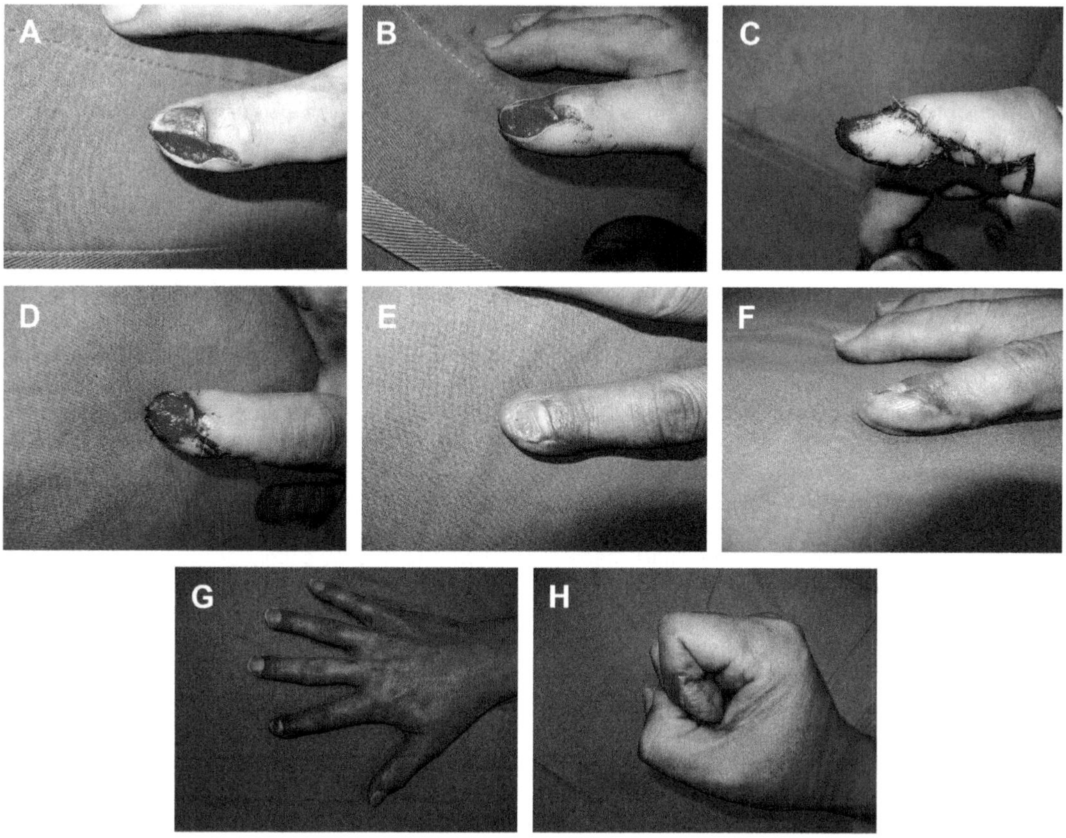

Fig. 1. (*A, B*) Right index finger tip oblique amputation with nail bed loss. (*C, D*) Reconstruction with homodigital neurovascular island flap based on the radial digital artery and nail bed transposition flap. (*E–H*) Results at 4 months with satisfactory pulp contour and motion.

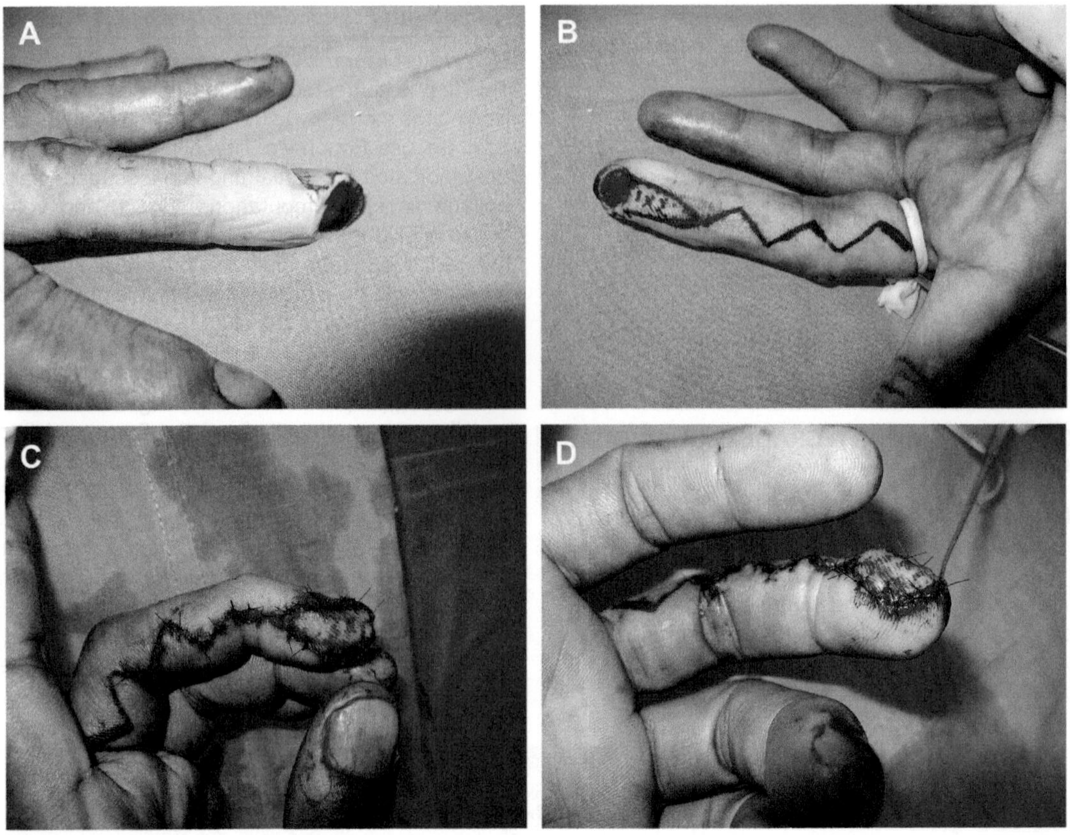

Fig. 2. (*A*) Oblique fingertip amputation of the left middle finger. (*B*) Long V-shaped flap and hemi-Bruner incision marked out. (*C*) The flap is advanced distally and inset distally first, then proximally. (*D*) The distal width of the flap matches the width of the defect.

A long V-shaped skin flap is marked out. The width of the flap distally corresponds to the width of the wound at the fingertip. The length of the flap is at least twice that of the width to better allow redistribution of the skin as the finger tapers toward its tip. A hemi-Bruner incision is first made at volar lateral side of the finger and the neurovascular bundle is identified at the proximal phalanx level and traced distally until it is seen to enter the marked out flap. Vascular branches of the proper digital artery are carefully ligated, especially the transverse branches at the neck of middle and proximal phalanx, to avoid tethering the flap. Dorsal branches of the proper digital artery must be ligated to increase the degree of flap advancement. Grayson and Cleland ligaments must be divided to adequately mobilize the pedicle. It is important to keep the digital nerve and artery together with a cuff of fat around the pedicle for venous drainage of the flap. Once the pedicle is freed proximally, the palmar margins of the flap are incised, and dissection proceeds straight down toward the flexor sheath. Care needs to be taken to include the pedicle in the flap and we suggest that the flap is raised completely off the flexor sheath, leaving no other tissue behind, in a palmar to lateral direction. Once the midaxial line of the digit has been reached, the dorsal skin margin of the flap is incised, and the flap completely islanded. The flap is then advanced and inset distally first before progressing proximally. The defect is closed in V-Y fashion and if deemed to be too tight, should be allowed to heal by secondary intention.

Flap advancement is possible because of the natural elasticity of the pedicle, surgical release of soft tissue tethers including branches of the digital arteries and Grayson and Cleland ligaments, and transposition of the pedicle toward the midline. Further advancement is facilitated by extending the incision into the palm and dissecting the pedicle to the common neurovascular bundle and mild flexion of the interphalangeal joints (IPJs) (**Fig. 3**). Larger defects involving most of the pulp skin unit are better resurfaced with options, such as the reverse vascular island or cross-finger flap (**Fig. 4**).

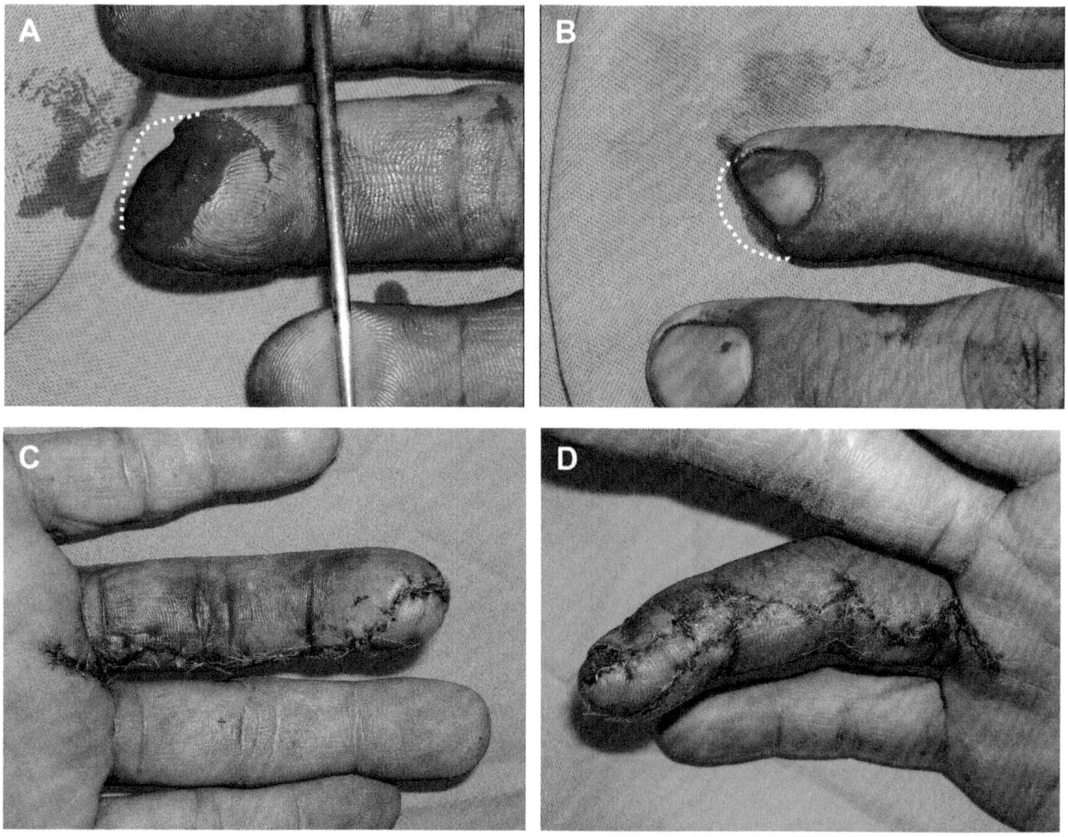

Fig. 3. (*A, B*) Slightly larger oblique amputations require more flap and pedicle advancement (*dotted white line* indicates advancement distance). (*C, D*) Mobilization of the neurovascular bundle to the junction of the common digital neurovascular bundle through a palm extension and slight finger flexion facilitates easy advancement.

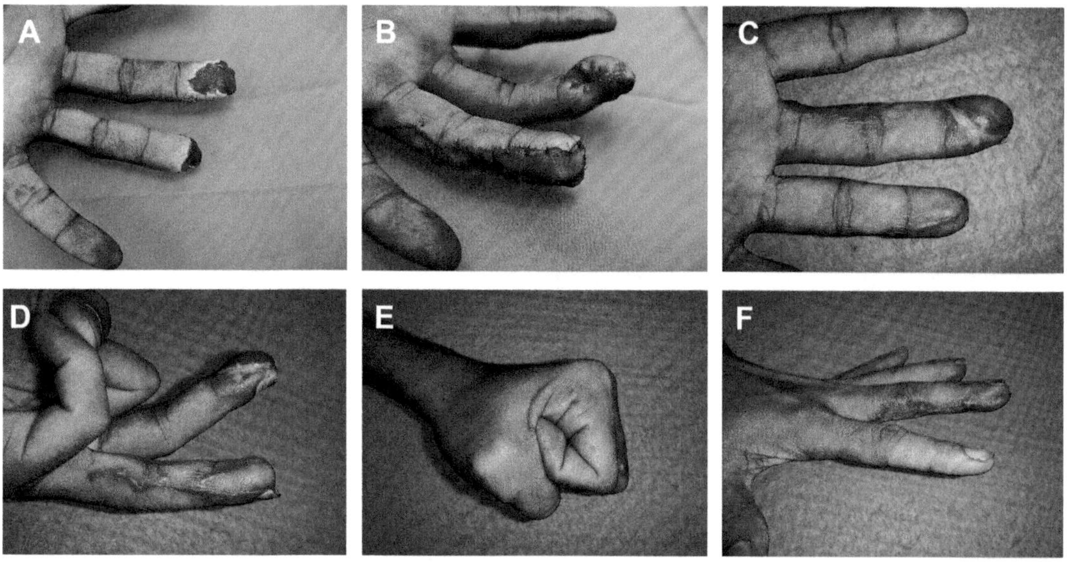

Fig. 4. (*A*) Large volar unfavorable fingertip loss of the middle finger and distal transverse fingertip loss of the ring finger. (*B*) Resurfacing with reverse vascular island flap for the middle finger and a homodigital neurovascular island advancement flap for the ring finger. (*C–F*) Cosmesis and function after 6 weeks.

Outcomes and complications In Foucher's series, 84% of patients recovered two-point discrimination between 3 and 7 mm and 60% between 3 and 5 mm. Foucher also reported total flap loss in 2 of 64 patients (3%) in his series and a mean proximal interphalangeal joint (PIPJ) contracture of 23° was present in 17% of the operated digits. Nakanishi and colleagues[16] found an average of 16° reduction in the passive extension angle of the PIPJ in patients after homodigital island flap. They found that old age, ulnar digit, and prolonged time for wound healing were significantly associated with PIPJ flexion contracture. Other complications include flap necrosis, cold intolerance, and a hook nail deformity from a tight distal inset and insufficient advancement.

Variation: pulp switch flap

In 1989, Foucher and colleagues[10] briefly described an "exchange-type" flap where the ulnar hemipulp is transferred as an island on to the radial hemipulp defect of the index finger. Elliot and colleagues[17] later described a side-to-side homodigital switch flap for the same purpose of restoring sensation in an insensate ulnar hemipulp of the thumb. In their three cases, the flap was not islanded but transposed with its radial digital neurovascular bundle. Silva and colleagues[18] reported their results in 16 cases, thumb and fingers included in which they also elevated a "pulp switch flap" based on the nondominant neurovascular bundle of a digit to resurface pulp loss on the dominant side of the digit. The largest mean defect size resurfaced was 2.85 cm^2 involving the thumb. All 16 flaps were islanded and transposed to cover the pulp defect and the donor defect was covered by a full-thickness hypothenar skin graft.

This concept is applied for coverage of critical defects over the dorsum of the digit from the distal interphalangeal joint to the PIPJ. In such instances, the flap is raised based solely on the digital artery preserving the digital nerve innervation of the finger pulp (**Fig. 5**). If the defect is small, an islanded digital artery flap is advanced to cover the defect without need for a skin graft (**Fig. 6**).

Outcomes and complications There were no instances of flap failure or loss in Silva's series. The two-point discrimination was 8 mm in the transposed pulps in all digits aside from the ring finger where it was 10 mm. Loss of motion was only noted in the little finger.

Heterodigital Island Flaps

Heterodigital neurovascular island flap

Since Moberg's and Littler's original description and Tubiana's elaboration of the technique, few modifications to the original description have been made. One such variation was described briefly by Hueston[19] in 1965. In his report, he reasoned that not just the hemipulp of the donor digit be elevated, but the entire skin proximal to that could be elevated as well to better provide for sensation to the thumb. He termed it the extended neurovascular island flap. In our

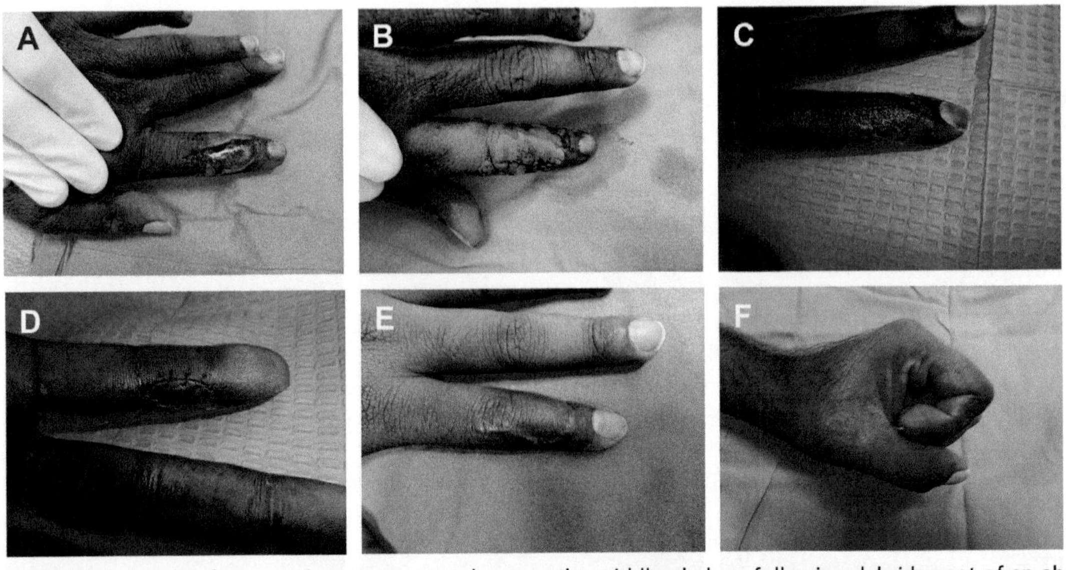

Fig. 5. (*A*) A dorsal defect exposing extensor tendon over the middle phalanx following debridement of an abscess. (*B*) Coverage with a transposition flap based on the ulnar digital artery. (*C, D*) Flap is well healed and viable at 2 weeks and full-thickness skin graft is well taken. (*E, F*) The thin flap sits well on the dorsum of the digit and motion is unimpeded in the digit.

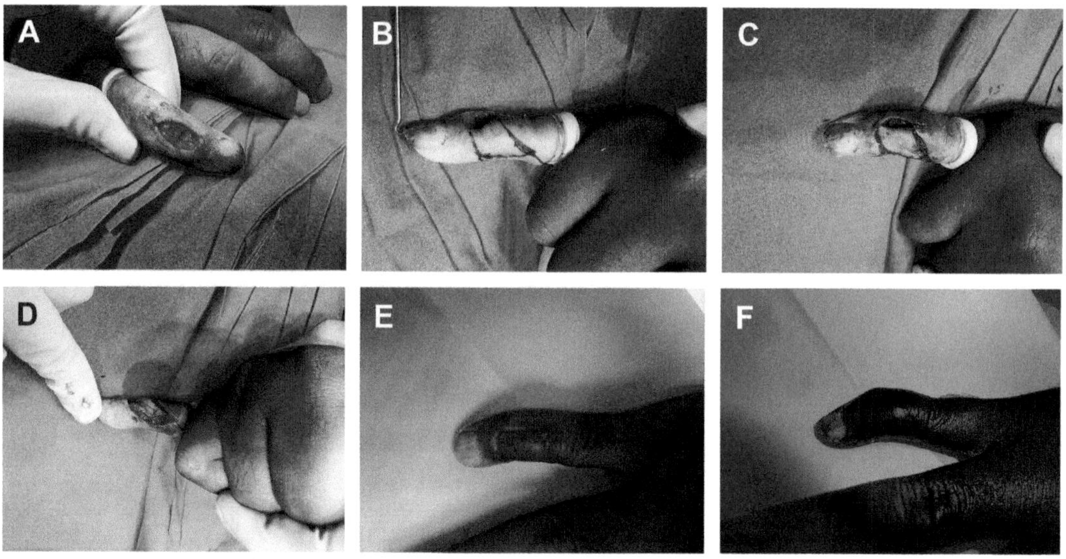

Fig. 6. (*A*) Septic arthritis of the distal interphalangeal joint of the small finger with tendon loss debrided until wound had a clean base and edges. (*B–D*) An island flap based on the ulnar digital artery is marked out, elevated, and advanced and transposed to cover the defect. The resultant donor wound is closed primarily. (*E, F*) The flap is well healed at 6 weeks and patient declined distal interphalangeal joint fusion because the digit was painless and functional.

practice, the heterodigital neurovascular island flap is reserved primarily for resurfacing thumb pulp loss, especially when homodigital options are not practical.

Operative technique The nondominant pulp of the donor finger should be chosen and in our practice, the ulnar hemipulp of the middle or index finger is preferred (**Fig. 7**). We prefer to avoid using the ulnar hemipulp of the ring finger because its digital neurovascular pedicle arises from the ulnar side of the palm and suffers from a shorter pedicle length when being transferred to the thumb. Furthermore, the cutaneous innervation is provided for by the ulnar nerve and may potentially contribute to poorer sensory cortical reorientation.

Patency of both digital arteries should be confirmed. The size of the defect is assessed, and a template created and marked out on the donor digit ulnar hemipulp. It is important that a reasonable amount of pulp skin is included in the flap to ensure better innervation of the flap. Brunauer incisions extending from the flap to the midpalm (Kaplan cardinal line) and from the thumb pulp defect to the base of the thumb are marked. The donor digit is first explored and the ulnar neurovascular bundle is identified in the region of the proximal phalanx and dissection then proceeds distally toward the flap and proximally to the midpalm. This ensures that digital nerve and artery are entering the flap.

It is crucial to avoid skeletonizing the pedicle because this increases the risk of disrupting the venae commitantes and the surrounding venules of the digital artery. The transverse retrotendinous communicating branches from the digital artery should be dissected and carefully ligated and the pedicle should be completely mobilized until the superficial palmar arch. At the branching point of the common digital artery, the other digital artery branch must be securely tied off while the digital nerve is further mobilized by interfascicular dissection of the common digital nerve with high-power loupe magnification or with the aid of a microscope.

The thumb is prepared by incising the palmar skin over the proximal phalanx of the thumb and elevating it as full-thickness flaps off the flexor pollicis sheath. A generous subcutaneous tunnel should be created between the base of the thumb and the midpalm incision. The palmar aponeurosis here should be carefully incised to avoid potential areas of constriction when the flap has been transferred.

Before islanding the flap, we place a vascular clamp on the pedicle proximally and release the arm tourniquet. This is to ensure that the rest of the digit remains perfused by the other digital artery. The flap is then islanded by dividing the neurovascular bundle exiting the flap distally and passed under the skin bridge to lie in the thumb pulp wound with care taken to avoid twisting the pedicle during this part of the procedure. Good hemostasis is essential to avoid the problems of hematoma formation and potential for

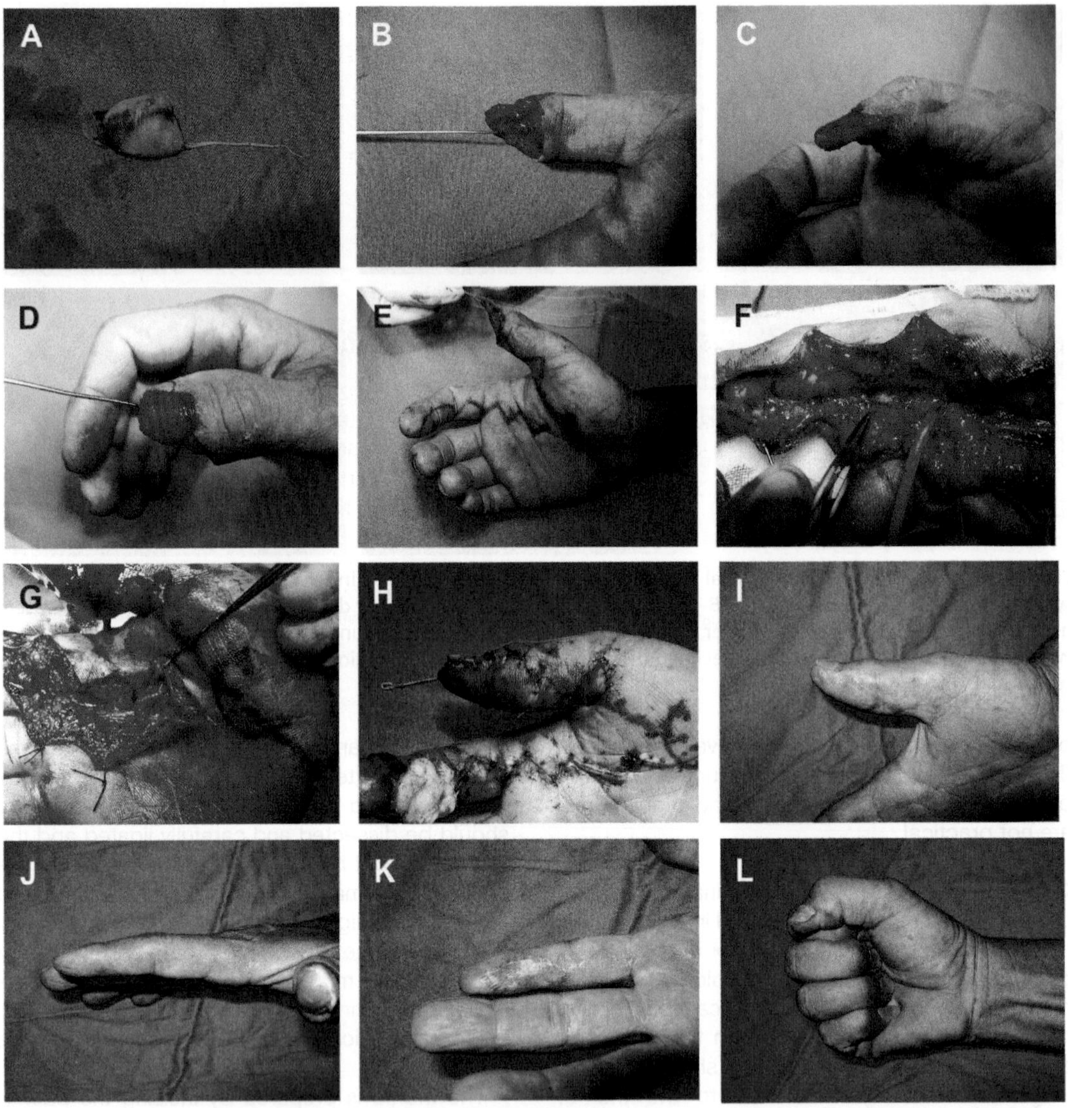

Fig. 7. (*A–D*) A large thumb pulp avulsion amputation that was found to have no suitable distal vessels in the amputate following exploration. (*E*) Flap dimensions marked out on the donor digit and planned surgical incisions. (*F*) The digital neurovascular bundle is dissected out maintaining some peribundle fat and tagged with an orange vessel loop. The retrotendinous communicating branches are marked with *black arrows*. (*G*) Dissection of the pedicle to the superficial palmar arch (*black arrow*) is crucial to avoid kinks in the artery when transferring. (*H*) Inset is completed with the thumb extended. (*I–L*) The result at 3 months is satisfactory with minimal loss of motion to the thumb or the donor digit. The pulp contour of the reconstructed thumb is slightly diminished because the resurfacing volume requirement cannot be completely fulfilled by this transfer.

compression of the neurovascular pedicle. The flap is then inset with the thumb fully extended. The donor defect is covered with a full-thickness skin graft harvested from the proximal medial forearm.

Variation: débranchment-rebranchment technique

To reduce the double sensibility phenomenon in the flap, De Conick[20] proposed transecting the digital nerve to the island flap and suturing it to the ulnar digital nerve of the thumb. Later on in 1981, Foucher and colleagues[21] described a similar technique named "débranchment-rebranchment" technique. The digital nerve to the flap is cut at two areas, proximally in the palm and distally near to the flap. The proximal end of the cut nerve is buried in the lumbrical muscle to avoid neuroma formation. The distal end of the digital nerve near to the flap is sutured to the ulnar digital nerve of the recipient thumb. A personal modification to this technique is harvesting the cutaneous branch to the palmar skin of a more lateral and proximally harvested flap and preserving the main trunk entering the pulp when resurfacing the radial hemipulp of the thumb (**Fig. 8**).

Variation: heterodigital arterialized flaps

In instances where sensory restoration is not critical, a heterodigital arterialized flap preserves the donor digit sensation while still conferring the benefits of a well-vascularized flap with a versatile reach (**Fig. 9**).[11] When larger flaps are required, a fasciocutaneous flap with the fascial extension harvested from the dorsum of the middle phalanx allows expansion of flap dimensions (**Fig. 10**A–J). In our practice, we preferentially harvest more of the dorsal skin and avoid the pulp skin because there is less of a resultant contour defect in the donor digit. Teoh and colleagues[14,15] modified the heterodigital arterialized island flap to include a dorsal subcutaneous vein to mitigate risk of venous congestion and flap complications. In our practice, we have not found this to be necessary.

Variation: heterodigital arterial flow-through flap

Wong and colleagues[22] reported the use of a heterodigital vascular island flap for simultaneous revascularization and soft tissue coverage in three patients. The distal end of the flap vessel was anastomosed to the distal digital artery stump of the devascularized or amputated finger to revascularize it. All three digits (two thumbs and one small finger) survived without any flap necrosis. This single-stage reconstructive procedure provides simultaneous arterial inflow and soft tissue coverage for finger injury with segmental vessel injuries (**Fig. 11**).

Outcomes and complications Sensory recovery of the flap is not always satisfactory and typically takes 6 to 12 months before cortical sensory reorientation occurs. Oka[23] compared two different

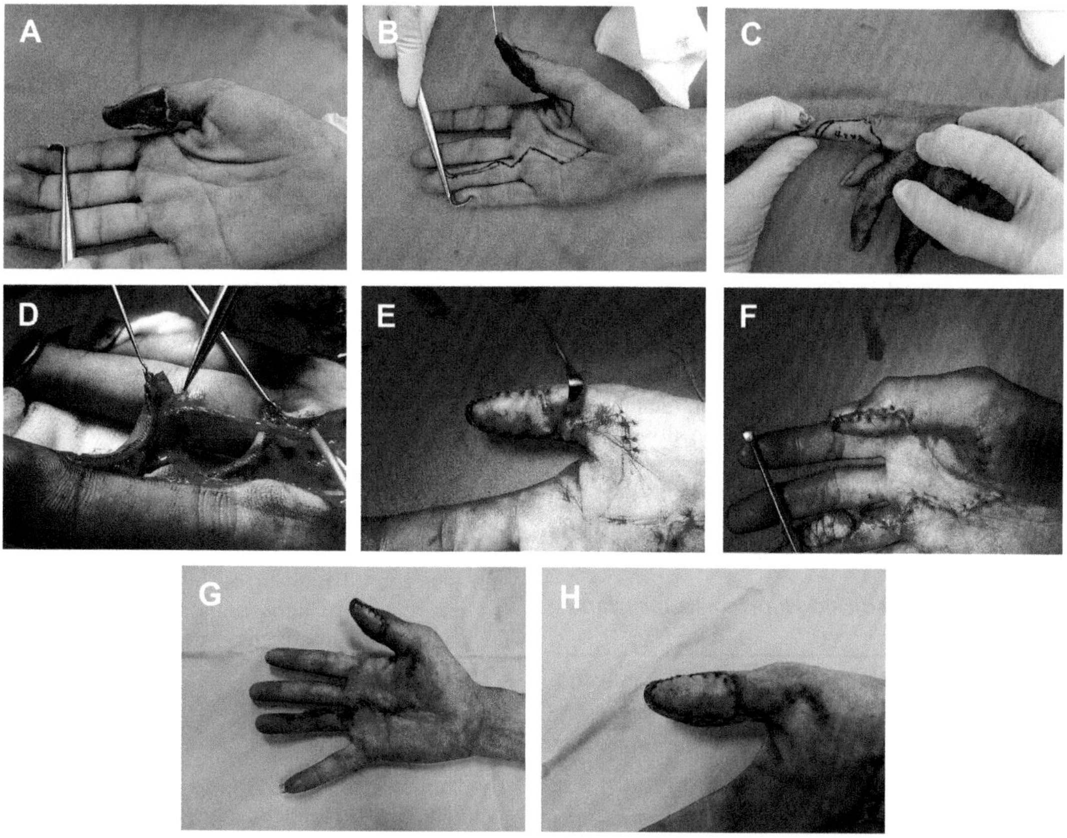

Fig. 8. (*A–C*) A predominantly radial pulp defect of the thumb is resurfaced by a heterodigital island flap from the ring finger, which is situated more laterally. (*D*) The cutaneous branch to the flap is identified (held by jeweler's forceps) and the flap is transferred based solely on the digital artery and its venae comitantes preserving the digital nerve proper to the pulp. (*E, F*) Flap immediately after coaptation of the nerve branch to the radial digital nerve of the thumb and inset. (*G, H*) Appearance after 2 weeks.

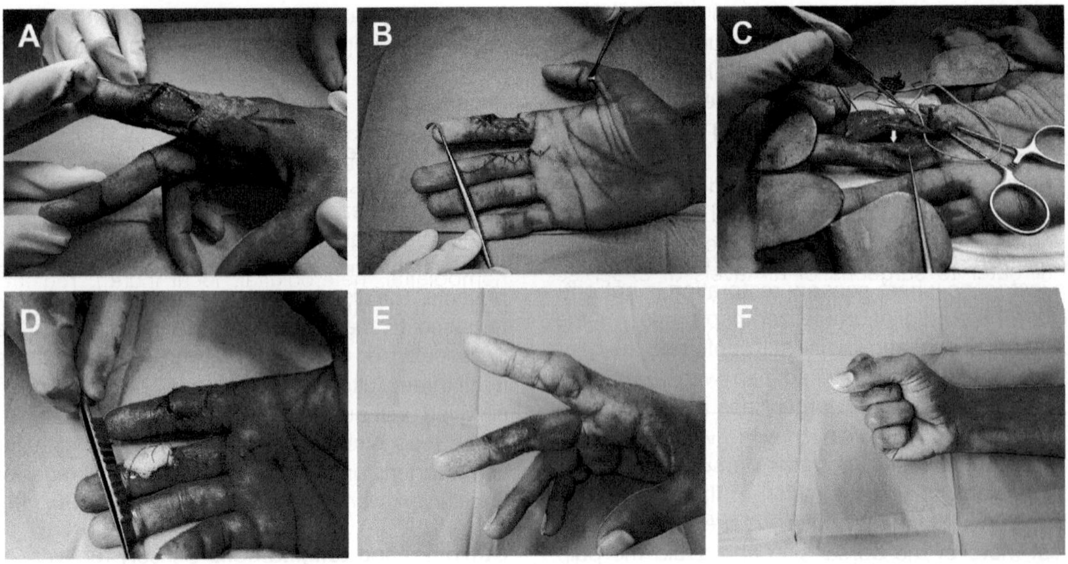

Fig. 9. (*A, B*) A moderate sized defect over the radial aspect of the index finger with exposed radial digital nerve is resurfaced by a heterodigital arterialized flap from the lateral and dorsal aspect of the adjacent middle finger based on its radial digital artery. (*C*) The flap is elevated on the digital artery with the dorsal digital nerve branch (*black arrow*) preserving the main digital nerve trunk (*white arrow*). In this patient, the branch of the ulnar digital artery of the index finger is preserved because the transfer distance is nearby (adjacent digit) and the radial digital artery of the index finger is nonviable. (*D–F*) Immediate postoperative appearance and at 6 months demonstrating excellent cosmesis and range of motion.

techniques and the sensory outcomes of both transfers. The first follows Moberg-Littler's classic description and the other a modification reported by Foucher and coworkers[21] in 1981 where the donor digital nerve is divided and sutured to the stump of the ulnar digital nerve in the thumb. All 21 flaps survived in Oka's series. However, he found that all patients had some degree of paresthesia and numbness in the thumb tip and had a mean two-point discrimination of approximately 9 mm. In the classic technique group, all nine patients experienced double sensation (thumb and donor digit) in the transferred island pulp and sensibility switching was only recognized in 60% of the tested times. In contrast, all 12 patients in the modified procedure group felt the flap as the thumb.

Homodigital Bipedicled Neurovascular Island Flap

In this group of flaps, the donor tissue is harvested from the injured digit, involving both neurovascular pedicles to provide a like-for-like sensate coverage.

Palmar advancement flap

Moberg originally described this bipedicled advancement flap to resurface the dennervated distal part of the thumb.[1] This flap is based on both neurovascular pedicles and the distance of advancement is approximately 1.5 cm.

Surgical anatomy The thumb has two arterial systems: a palmar and dorsal system. The two palmar digital arteries most frequently arise from princeps pollicis artery, and in 10% of the cases immediately from the superficial palmar arch, or from the deep palmar arch. The dorsal system is composed of an ulnar and radial dorsal artery arising from the first dorsal metacarpal artery in the former and the latter smaller vessel from the radial artery in the anatomic snuff box. This distinct dorsal arterial system allows the bipedicled elevation of the palmar skin of the thumb without leading to vascular embarrassment.

Operative technique The flap is suited for transverse thumb tip amputations, which are small and less than 1.5 cm in length. In our practice, we use this flap incorporating Kojima and coworker's[24] V-Y modification but reserve this flap principally for the thumb.

The flap is designed with two parallel midlateral incisions that extend from the wound to the palmodigital crease terminating in a V-shaped incision. The flap is dissected off the flexor tendon sheath, including both neurovascular pedicles within the flap. Only Cleland ligament needs to be divided to allow mobilization of the flap. After this maneuver, the flap is carefully raised from distal to proximal until the proximal V incision. An attempt should be made to preserve the dorsal branches

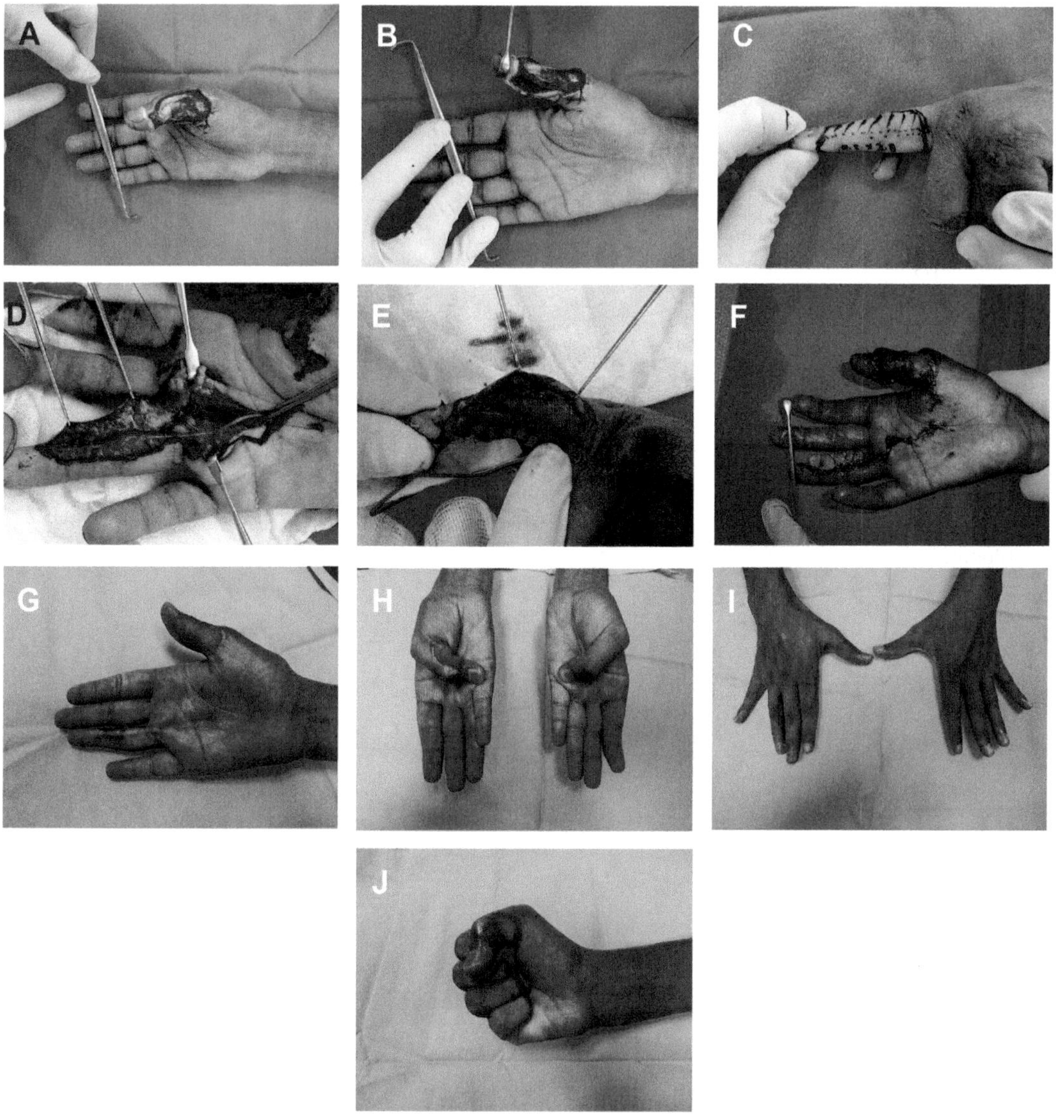

Fig. 10. (*A, B*) Large area of skin loss over the dorsal-lateral and volar radial aspect of the thumb from infection exposing tendon and radial digital nerve. (*C*) A large heterodigital arterialized flap is marked out according to the dimensions of the defect. The *hatched lines* representing the fascial extension. (*D*) The donor digital nerve is dissected and skeletonized to preserve the venous supply of the arterial pedicle. (*E*) The dorsal skin at the margin of the *hatched line* is elevated thinly to preserve the subcutaneous fascia, which is elevated off the paratenon of the extensors. (*F*) The fascial extension is covered with a split-thickness skin graft. (*G–J*) Functional result and appearance after 4 months demonstrating excellent motion and cosmesis of donor digit and recipient thumb.

from the palmar digital arteries to supplement the dorsal circulation and to avoid dorsal skin necrosis. If the dorsal arteries must be ligated to facilitate flap advancement, the pedicles should be clamped with microvascular clamps to ascertain an adequate dorsal circulation before these vessels are divided. The flap is then advanced distally until the critical defect at the fingertip is adequately covered. The degree of advancement is facilitated by the V-Y closure proximally and is further increased by flexion at the IPJ during flap inset (**Fig. 12**).

Outcomes and complications Foucher and colleagues[25] reported successful flap elevation and survival in 13 patients with distal thumb injuries. In their series, there were no instances of IPJ flexion contracture and cold intolerance seemed to be the main problem. Sensibility and padding at the tip of the reconstructed thumb was deemed

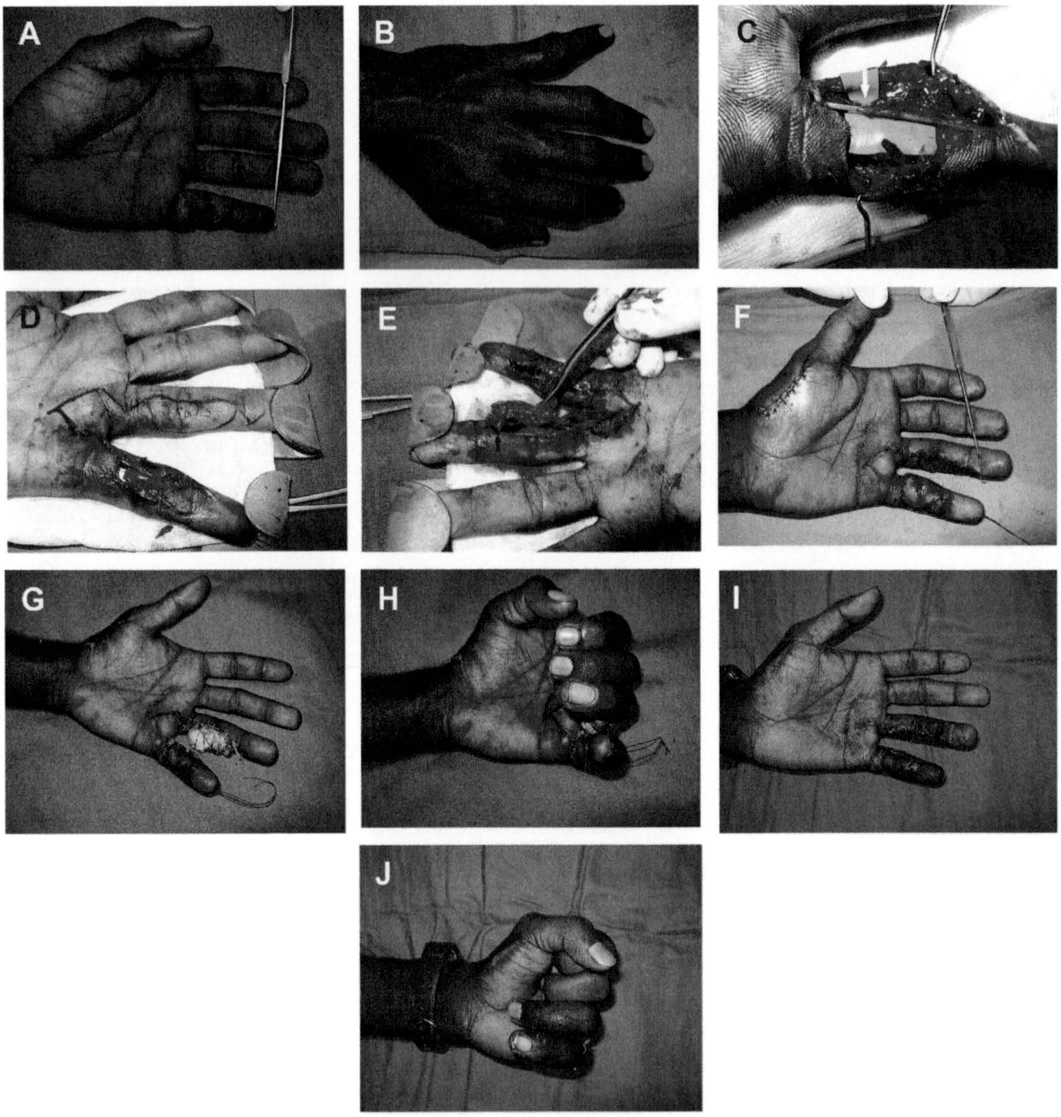

Fig. 11. (*A, B*) A crush injury with a proximal phalanx fracture and critical arterial injury. The pulp of the little finger is dusky. (*C*) The radial digital artery (*white arrow*) is thrombosed and the ulnar digital artery is ruptured (*black arrow*) with proximal vessel contusion. (*D, E*) After preparation of the vessels, the size of the wound is assessed and templated on the ulnar side of the ring finger (*D*). The vascular island flap is elevated preserving the digital nerve (*E*) in the donor; when doing so, a longer distal stump is preferred (*black arrow*). (*F*) Immediate pinking of the pulp and flap following microvascular anastomosis and flap inset. (*G, H*) Fingertip and flap viability at Day 5. (*I, J*) Flap viability and motion recovery 1-month postsurgery.

to be excellent in this series, although lateral instability of the pulp was a problem in a few patients. Kojima and colleagues[24] reported successful flap elevation and survival in 14 fingers with an advancement of 10 to 15 mm. They were careful to maintain two to four dorsal arterial branches of each digital artery during flap elevation and advancement. No complications were reported in their series.

The main complication of this technique is an IPJ flexion contracture, flap necrosis at the distal end from tight inset, and the risk of dorsal skin necrosis if care is not taken to preserve the dorsal branches of the digital arteries.[26,27]

AUTHORS' PREFERENCE

Homodigital Island Flap

Our preference for using this technique is for resurfacing small oblique fingertip amputations using a neurovascular island flap. An advancement distance of 15 mm is easily accomplished and further

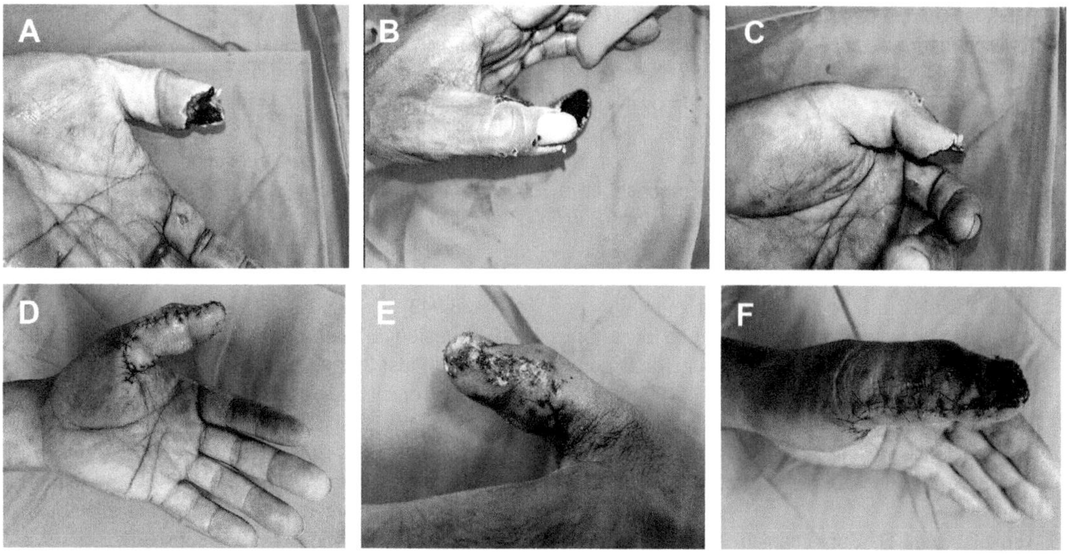

Fig. 12. (*A–C*) Thumb tip pulp loss for crush amputation. (*D–F*) Five days after bipedicled palmar advancement flap with proximal V-Y closure.

advancement is possible by dissection of the pedicle proximal to the digitopalmar crease. For small critical defects over the dorsum of the middle phalanx, we elect to use the antegrade flow digital artery island flap based on the pulp switch concept, limiting morbidity to the same digit. We reserve the pulp switch flap for instances where a long radial hemipulp defect of the index or middle finger needs resurfacing.

Heterodigital Island Flap

We perform the heterodigital neurovascular island flap mainly for resurfacing thumb pulp loss that is medium sized and long, in particular when the ulnar hemipulp is deficient. When the entire thumb pulp unit is lost, we offer patients a free toe pulp transfer. Patients who decline this option usually require a heterodigital neurovascular island flap with dorsal cutaneous or fascial extensions to cover the entire thumb pulp. The heterodigital arterialized flap is our preferred option when there are medium to large (up to 4×3 cm) defects of a digit. In these instances, using a fascial extension reduces donor morbidity. This flap has great versatility and is used to resurface skin defects in the palm or dorsum of the hand. It is used also as a flow-through flap and is an attractive single-stage reconstructive option in those uncommon scenarios where soft tissue loss and critical arterial injury are present.

Homodigital Bipedicled Island Flap

Our preference is to use this flap for transverse thumb tip amputations not exceeding 15 mm in advancement length and incorporating Kojima's V-Y advancement modification for the proximal tail. Although authors have described the use of this flap successfully for the fingers, we believe there are other resurfacing options that require less dissection and suffer less from the potential of dorsal skin necrosis in the finger.

SUMMARY

Antegrade flow digital artery flaps offer a versatile single-stage reconstructive option for defects in the same digit the flap is elevated or for distant digits and parts of the hand with the advantage of being sensate when the digital nerve is included. When used for thumb pulp reconstruction, disconnecting the digital nerve of the pedicle proximally and neurorrhaphy to the ulnar digital nerve of the thumb is recommended. The main complication from homodigital flaps is a contracture consequent to excessive advancement and flexion of the IPJ. Venous congestion in heterodigital flaps is avoided by careful pedicle dissection and preservation of perivascular venules and venae comitantes.

REFERENCES

1. Moberg E. Discussion on Brooks D. The place of nerve-grafting in orthopaedic surgery. J Bone Joint Surg Am 1955;37A(2):299–326.
2. Littler JW. Neurovascular pedicle transfer of tissue in reconstructive surgery of the hand. J Bone Joint Surg 1956;38A:4–917.

3. Tubiana R, Duparc J. Restoration of sensibility in the hand by neurovascular skin island transfer. J Bone Joint Surg 1961;43B(3):474–80.
4. Peacock FE. Reconstruction of the hand by the local transfer of composite tissue island flaps. Plast Reconstr Surg 1960;25(4):298–311.
5. Moberg E. Aspects of sensation in reconstructive surgery in the upper extremity. J Bone Joint Surg 1964;46A(4):817–25.
6. O'Brien B. Neurovascular pedicle transfers in the hand. Aust N Z J Surg 1965;35:1–11.
7. Joshi BB. A local dorsolateral island flap for restoration of sensation after avulsion injury of fingertip pulp. Plast Reconstr Surg 1974;54:175–82.
8. Pho RW. Restoration of sensation using a local neurovascular island flap as a primary procedure in extensive pulp loss of the fingertip. Injury 1975;8:20–4.
9. Venkataswami R, Subramaniam N. Oblique triangular flap: a new method of repair for oblique amputations of fingertip and thumb. Plast Reconstr Surg 1980;66(2):296–300.
10. Foucher G, Smith D, Penpinello C, et al. Homodigital neurovascular island flaps for digital pulp loss. J Hand Surg Br 1989;14B:204–8.
11. Rose EH. Local arterialized island flap coverage of difficult hand defects preserving donor digit sensibility. Plast Reconstr Surg 1983;72(6):848–57.
12. Tsai TM, Yuen C. A neurovascular island flap for volar-oblique fingertip amputations. J Hand Surg Br 1996;21B(1):94–8.
13. Lim GJS, Yam AKT, Lee JYL, et al. The spiral flap for fingertip resurfacing: short-term and long-term results. J Hand Surg 2008;33A:340–7.
14. Teoh LC, Tay SC, Yong FC, et al. Heterodigital arterialized flaps for large finger wounds: results an indications. Plast Reconstr Surg 2003;111:1905.
15. Tay SC, Teoh LC, Tan SH, et al. Extending the reach of the heterodigital arterialized flap by vein division and repair. Plast Reconstr Surg 2004;114:1450.
16. Nakanishi A, Omokawa S, Iida A, et al. Predictors of proximal interphalangeal joint flexion contracture after homodigital island flap. J Hand Surg Am 2015;40(11):2155–9.
17. Elliot D, Southgate CM, Staiano JJ. A homodigital switch flap to restore sensation to the ulnar border of the thumb. J Hand Surg Br 2003;28B:409–13.
18. Silva JB, Pires FK, Teixeira LF. The pulp switch flap: an option for the treatment of loss of the dominant half of the digital pulp. J Hand Surg Eur Vol 2013;38:948–51.
19. Hueston J. The extended neurovascular island flap. Br J Plast Surg 1965;18:304–5.
20. De Conick A. Transplantation hétéro-digitale avec réinnervation locale. Acta Orthop Belg 1975;31(2):170–6.
21. Foucher G, Braun FM, Merle M, et al. La technique du "débranchment-rebranchment" due lambear en ilot pédiculé. Ann Chir 1981;35(4):301–3.
22. Wong MZ, Tan DMK, Sebastin SJ, et al. Heterodigital vascular island flap for simultaneous resurfacing and revascularization of digits. Ann Plast Surg 2009;62:34–7.
23. Oka Y. Sensory function of the neurovascular island flap in thumb reconstruction: comparison of original and modified procedures. J Hand Surg Am 2000;25(4):637–43.
24. Kojima T, Kinoshita Y, Hirase Y, et al. Extended palmar advancement flap with V-Y closure for finger injuries. Br J Plast Surg 1994;47:275–9.
25. Foucher G, Deleaere O, Citron N, et al. Long-term outcome of neurovascular palmar advancement flaps for distal thumb injuries. Br J Plast Surg 1999;52:64–8.
26. Snow JW. The use of a volar flap for repair of fingertip amputations: a preliminary report. Plast Reconstr Surg 1967;40(2):163–8.
27. Shaw MH. Neurovascular island pedicled flaps for terminal digit scars: a hazard. Br J Plast Surg 1971;24:161–5.

Retrograde Flow Digital Artery Flaps

Benjamin Zhi Qiang Seah, MB, BS,
Sandeep J. Sebastin, MCh (Plastic Surgery), MMed (Surgery), FAMS (Hand Surgery)*,
Alphonsus Khin Sze Chong, MBBS, MRCS

KEYWORDS

• Retrograde flow • Digital artery flaps • Digital defects

KEY POINTS

- Retrograde flow digital artery flaps are a versatile single-stage option for the coverage of fingertip and dorsal digital defects.
- Techniques vary predominantly in the tissue incorporated (adipofascial or cutaneous) and the inclusion of the digital nerve or its branches in the pedicle with subsequent neurorrhaphy.
- Complications include venous congestion, flexion contracture, and cold intolerance.

INTRODUCTION

The concept and utility of a retrograde flow digital artery island flap using the anastomotic network between the 2 proper digital arteries was introduced by Weeks and Wray in 1973.[1] They demonstrated how a retrograde flow digital artery flap raised on the ulnolateral border of the proximal phalanx could be used for coverage of a dorsal proximal interphalangeal joint (PIPJ) defect.

There are several advantages associated with retrograde flow digital artery flaps:

1. A long distally based vascular pedicle with a wide arc of rotation (up to 180°) effectively means that the flap can be used to cover any defect located from the proximal phalanx to the fingertip. This also means that digit length can be preserved to a large extent, minimizing the disabilities associated with digit shortening.
2. A large flap surface area of up to 8.0 cm^2 (4.0 cm × 2.0 cm)[2] means that significant pulp loss or digit defects can be adequately resurfaced in a like-for-like fashion with glabrous skin.
3. The thin, flexible, and durable nature of the flap, coupled with the reliability and robustness of the arterial supply as long as both digital arteries and the distal arterial arch providing reverse arterial perfusion is patent, means that the risk of flap failure is low.
4. Donor site morbidity is minimal because the grafted donor site on the lateral aspect of the digit is relatively hidden. Furthermore, the flap is typically raised from the injured digit itself. This keeps the morbidity to the injured digit and limits impact of the reconstruction on other unaffected digits.
5. The possibility of a concomitant neurorrhaphy to create a sensible flap lends significant value especially in the context of fingertip reconstruction.
6. This single-stage reconstruction, together with a localized operative field, offers the benefits of faster recovery, minimal immobilization, quicker progression to rehabilitation, redundancy of cortical reeducation of the recipient site, lower cost, and shorter hospitalization.

HISTORICAL REVIEW

The concept of the retrograde flow digital artery flap is a result of detailed anatomic studies (**Table 1**) that identified transverse anastomoses between

Disclosure: None.
Department of Hand & Reconstructive Microsurgery, National University Health System, Tower Block, Level 11, 1E Kent Ridge Road, Singapore 119228
* Corresponding author.
E-mail address: sandeep_sebastin@nuhs.edu.sg

Hand Clin 36 (2020) 47–56
https://doi.org/10.1016/j.hcl.2019.08.005

Table 1
Key time points in understanding the arterial system of the finger relevant to retrograde flaps

Author(s), Year	Description
Yamamoto,[3] 1939	Deep arcuate anastomosis at approximately the midpoint of both the middle and proximal phalanges. Anastomosis across the proximal phalanx is predominant over that in the middle phalanx
Saito,[4] 1956	Commissural (anastomotic) branches occur mostly in pairs and that large branches coincide at the levels of the proximal interphalangeal and distal interphalangeal joints
Edwards,[5] 1960	Called these anastomotic branches the proximal and distal transverse digital arteries and reported that such arteries are constantly present at the level of the neck of the phalanx in contact with the phalangeal bone
Zbrodowski et al,[6] 1981	Named these anastomotic branches the digitopalmar arch
Cormack & Lamberty,[7] 1986	In the thumb, the dorsal skin branch arises from the palmar digital artery level with the center of the proximal phalanx and runs dorsally and distally to anastomose with the distal arcades. This anatomic pattern allows the homodigital flap to be raised without sacrificing the digital artery, and it is perfused by reverse flow through these distal arcades
Strauch & de Moura,[8] 1990	Described 4 dorsal branches of the proper palmar digital artery in each phalanx with the dorsal cutaneous branch and the cutaneous branch from the transverse palmar arch supplying the dorsum of the finger. Described 3 constant major palmar arches in each digit: the proximal and middle arches in association with the C1 and C3 pulleys, and the distal arch just distal to the FDP insertion
Kojima et al,[9] 1990	The digital palmar arch arises in the proximal two-thirds of the proximal phalanx and lies halfway along the middle phalanx. It perforates the deepest part of the side of the flexor tendon sheath to lie beneath the check rein ligament of the volar plate and passes between the posterior wall of the tendon sheath and the periosteum to form the arch

Data from Refs.[3–9]

the radial and ulnar digital arteries. There are 3 major anastomoses across the length of the finger, namely, the proximal, middle, and distal transverse arch. The proximal arch is located at the level of the C1 pulley, the middle arch at the level of the C3 pulley, and the distal arch immediately distal to the insertion of the flexor digitorum profundus (FDP) tendon. There are also 3 arcades in the distal phalanx: the superficial arcade, the proximal subungual arcade, and the distal subungual arcade. These arcades are interconnected and form a particularly rich vascular plexus in the nail bed and the terminal segment of the finger. The appreciation of the constant dorsal branches of the proper palmar digital artery in each phalanx supplying the dorsolateral skin of the phalanx enabled reverse pedicle island flaps to be raised not only off the proximal phalanx but also off the middle phalanx and thumb (see **Table 1**). The evolution and modifications to the retrograde flow digital artery flap since its introduction are summarized in **Table 2**. Following success associated with the homodigital reverse vascular island flap, neurotization of the digital nerve or its branches to the ends of the digital nerve in the stump allowed the possibility of making this flap sensate.

PREREQUISITES AND INDICATIONS

The patency of both digital arteries along with a patent middle transverse anastomotic arch at the level of the C3 pulley (neck of middle phalanx) providing reverse arterial perfusion of the flap is critical to the success of the retrograde flow digital artery flap. In theory, the patency of the digital arteries can be checked by a digital Allen test before surgery. However, in practice, it is difficult to perform a digital Allen test in a patient with pulp loss. The authors determine the adequacy of perfusion of the flap and the finger by placing a vessel clamp across the digital artery after islanding the flap and then releasing the tourniquet. The integrity and suitability of the donor site should also be considered. The homodigital reverse

Table 2
Timeline describing the evolution and modifications to the retrograde flow digital artery flap

Author(s), Year	Description
Weeks & Wray,[1] 1973	Distally based digital artery flap for coverage of a dorsal PIPJ defect
Brunelli,[10] 1987	Homodigital reverse neurovascular island flap
Oberlin et al,[11] 1988	Homodigital reverse vascular island flap for coverage of large defects over the middle phalanx and distal interphalangeal joint
Lai et al,[2] 1989	Homodigital reverse digital artery flap for fingertip reconstruction; 11 patients, including 10 with fingertip defects and 1 with a volar defect of the middle phalanx
Kojima et al,[9] 1990	Homodigital reverse vascular pedicle digital island flap; 8 fingers (7 patients), of which 6 pulp defects, 1 amputated stump, and 1 fingertip defect
Brunelli & Mathoulin,[12] 1991	Homodigital reverse neurovascular island flap for sensible coverage of large finger pulp defects
Endo et al,[13] 1992	Homodigital reverse neurovascular island flap using dorsal digital nerve and proper palmar digital artery as a retrograde vascular pedicle; 3 patients
Lai et al,[14] 1993	Homodigital reverse neurovascular island flap innervated through bilateral neurorrhaphy involving both the dorsal branch from the proper digital nerve and the superficial sensory branch from the corresponding radial or ulnar nerve; 3 cases of pulp defects
Sapp et al,[15] 1993	Homodigital reverse digital artery island flap; 13 flaps (11 patients)
Niranjan & Armstrong[16] 1994	Homodigital reverse vascular island flap for repair of volar or dorsal tissue loss on the finger or thumb; 25 cases, including 5 thumbs with distal phalangeal defects
Bene et al,[17] 1994	Homodigital reverse dorsal digital island flap based on the dorsal digital artery
Leupin et al,[18] 1997	Dorsal middle phalangeal finger flap, (neuro)vascular island flap based on a palmar proper digital artery, its venae comitantes (and/or a separate dorsal vein), and the dorsal branch(es) of the palmar digital nerve; 43 flaps (3 retrograde)
Germann et al,[19] 1997	Heterodigital reverse cross finger island flap; 5 patients
Adani et al,[20] 1999	Heterodigital reverse neurovascular island flap; 6 patients
Karacalar et al,[21] 2000	Homodigital reverse neurovascular island flap incorporating the proper digital nerve
Chang et al,[22] 2005	Homodigital reverse digital adipofascial flap; 8 patients
Li & Cui,[23] 2005	Homodigital reverse neurovascular island flap based on the end dorsal branch of the digital artery

Data from Refs.[1,2,9–23]

vascular island flap based on the proper digital artery is useful in the reconstruction of large pulp defects, dorsal and lateral defects of the distal phalanx, the distal interphalangeal joint, middle phalanx, and up to the PIPJ. For finger pulp defects, sensory restoration by means of neurorrhaphy involving either the proper digital nerve or its branches can be attempted.

SURGICAL ANATOMY

The arterial supply for this flap is by reverse flow into the digital artery via the middle transverse anastomotic arch located at the level of the neck of the middle phalanx in relation to the C3 pulley. Although the distal transverse arch distal to the FDP insertion and the subungual arcades can also provide flow into the divided digital artery, these anastomoses are usually in the zone of injury in a patient with pulp loss. The digital artery does not follow a straight line from proximal to distal but varies in its depth at different locations along the finger. It is in a relatively deeper plane at the mid-shaft and neck of the proximal phalanx, becomes more superficial near the PIPJ, and becomes deeper again near the mid-shaft of the

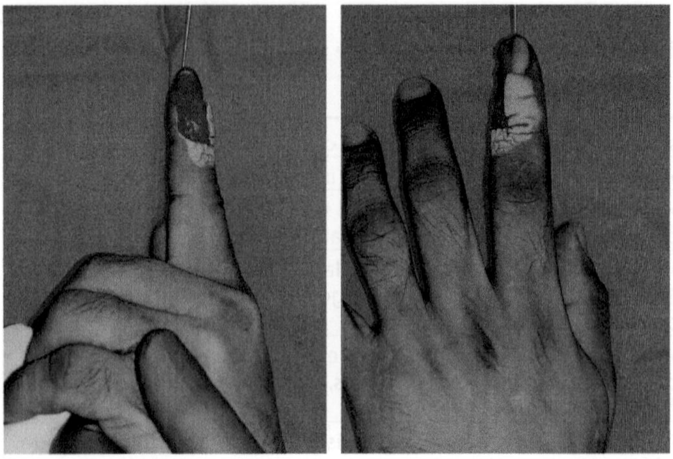

Fig. 1. Traumatic loss of ulnar hemipulp of right index finger.

middle phalanx. The venous return is via the adventitial venules within the vasa vasorum. The return has to occur against the direction of flow, and these small veins/venules struggle to drain the inflow via the digital artery. These factors are responsible for the high incidence of venous congestion associated with this flap. The flap is typically designed over the dorsolateral aspect of proximal phalanx. The proper digital nerve passes along one edge of the flap, but the innervation to this area of the skin is by the dorsal branch of the proper digital nerve that arises in the palm. In order to make this flap sensate, the dorsal branch needs to be identified proximal to the flap, included within the flap, and a repair performed to a suitable proper digital nerve in the pulp.

OPERATIVE TECHNIQUE

This flap typically requires 60 to 90 minutes to complete, including 30 to 45 minutes of tourniquet time, and can be challenging for beginners to perform under local anesthesia. The patient is administered regional or general anesthesia and positioned supine with the arm supported on a hand table. The size and shape of the defect (**Fig. 1**) are outlined, and the flap is designed in accordance with the required dimensions (**Fig. 2**). The flap is centered over the dorsolateral aspect of the proximal phalanx. The authors' preference is to limit the flap to non-contact areas of the digits, that is, ulnar aspect of the index, long, and ring fingers, and radial aspect of the little finger. The flap should be designed such that it avoids the "U"-shaped web fold to prevent development of a flexion contracture. One of the senior authors (S.J.S.) designs his reverse vascular island flap like a "speech balloon," that is, an ellipse with a triangular extension that points dorsally (see **Fig. 2**). Once the flap is rotated, the triangular extension overlies the vascular pedicle in the bridge segment between the defect and the flap donor site and allows closure of the bridge segment without constricting the underlying vascular pedicle.

A zig-zag hemi-Bruner incision is designed along the longitudinal axis of the pedicle. The

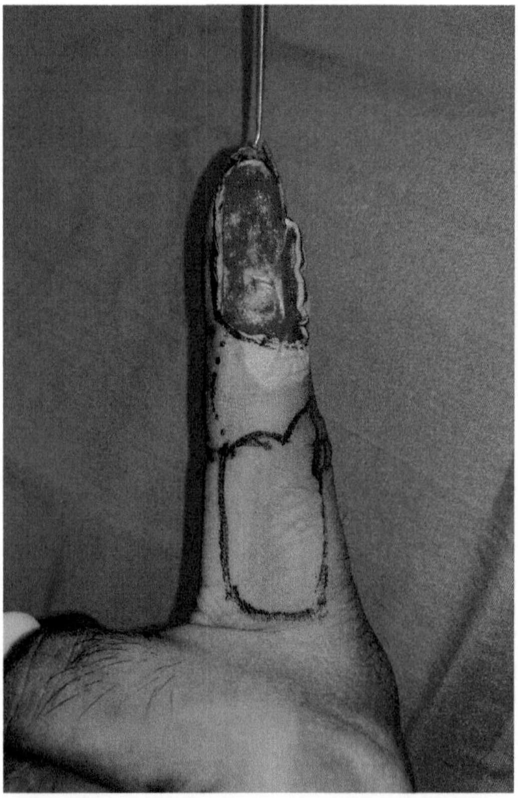

Fig. 2. Design of the flap on dorsoulnar surface incorporating the "speech balloon" pointing dorsally.

skin incision is made in the proximal region of the flap, and the neurovascular bundle is exposed by dividing Grayson ligament. The flap is subsequently elevated in a proximal-to-distal and anterior-to-posterior direction. The digital nerve is identified and mobilized toward the midline, keeping all the soft tissue and its perivascular sleeve of adipose tissue containing the delicate concomitant veins that provide venous drainage for the flap along with the digital artery. This requires division of the branches of the digital nerve going laterally. It is important not to take too much fat with the flap especially at the margins of the flap. The flap can become quite swollen in the postoperative period, and taking too much fat will make inset difficult (**Fig. 3**). Only enough fat to keep the digital artery in continuity with the overlying skin is required. The vessel is elevated superficial to the flexor sheath and the extensor tendon paratenon. The vascular pedicle should not be dissected beyond the midpoint of the middle phalanx to avoid compromising the transverse anastomosis situated at the neck of the middle phalanx.

The skin between the pulp defect and the distal end of pedicle dissection is opened in a subdermal plane to avoid injuring the deeper anastomotic vessels. It is important to complete all dissection before tourniquet release because dissection after tourniquet release runs a risk of injuring the tenuous venous drainage as well as the transverse anastomotic branches.

The proximal digital artery is temporarily occluded with a vessel clamp; the tourniquet is released, and finger and flap perfusion is confirmed (**Fig. 4**). Subsequently, hemostasis is achieved, and the digital artery is ligated proximally. The flap is then rotated up to 180° into the defect and inset (**Fig. 5**). To prevent compression of the vascular pedicle in the bridge segment, one can either use the "speech balloon" flap design (see **Fig. 2**) or apply a small skin graft over the vascular pedicle (**Fig. 6**).[2] The donor site is covered with a full-thickness skin graft (see **Fig. 5**). One of the senior authors (S.J.S.) no longer uses a tie-over dressing for the skin graft and begins mobilizing the finger on the second postoperative day (**Fig. 7**).

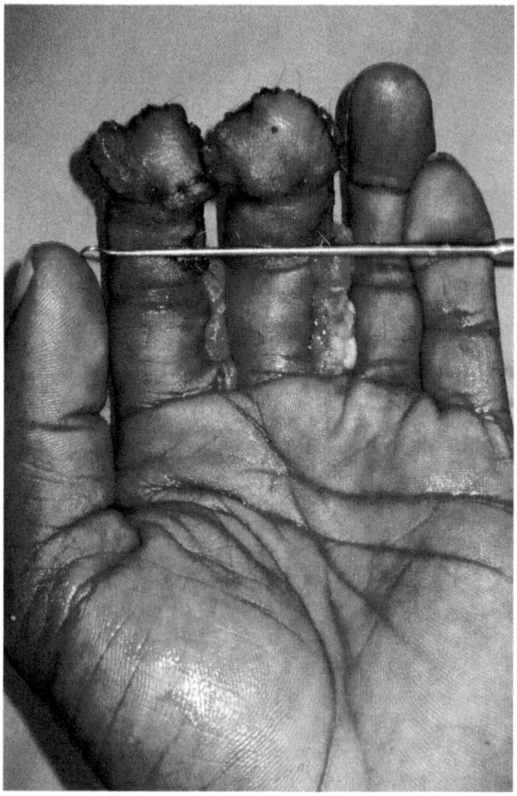

Fig. 3. Two retrograde flow digital artery flaps for pulp loss of middle and index fingers. Note that the flaps have been elevated with a large amount of fat, making inset difficult.

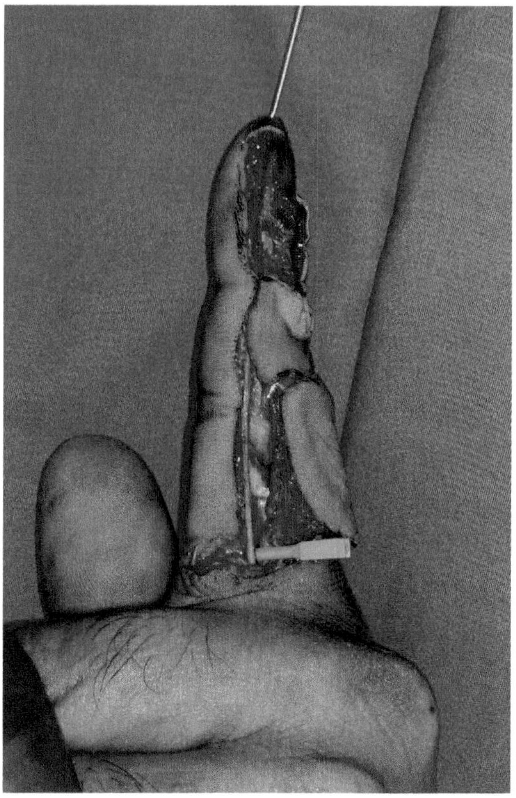

Fig. 4. Flap elevation for patient depicted in **Figs. 1** and **2** completed with vascular clamp in position before release of tourniquet to confirm perfusion of the finger and flap.

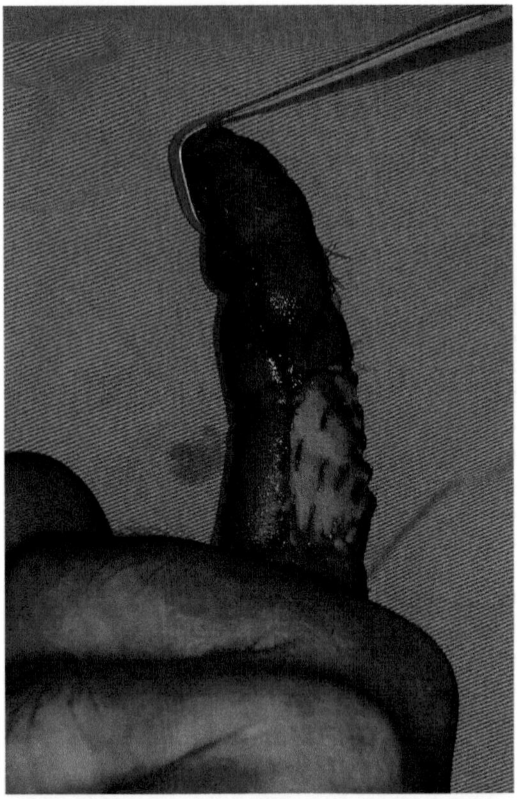

Fig. 5. Flap inset. Note position of "speech balloon" to prevent compression of vascular pedicle in the bridge segment and full-thickness skin graft to cover donor defect.

VARIATIONS

The variations of the retrograde flow digital artery flap include the adipofascial flap, neurovascular flap, cross finger flap, and the heterodigital flap. The adipofascial flap was described by Chang and colleagues[22] in 2005. The main advantages of this variation are that the donor site can be closed linearly and skin grafting is not required. However, the recipient site requires a skin graft. Chang and colleagues used this technique in 8 patients (6 with fingertip loss, one with dorsal loss, and one with a dorsal defect after tumor excision). No flap necrosis was observed; donor site morbidity was minimal, and no note-worthy motion limitation during the follow-up period of at least 6 months was present.

The neurovascular variation of this flap was described by Karacalar and colleagues[21] in 2000. In this variation, the proper digital nerve is divided and included within the flap. The divided end of the nerve is then sutured to one of the digital nerves in the pulp to restore sensation. The main benefit of harvesting the nerve is that elevating the artery and the nerve together allows more perineurovascular fat to be included within the flap, ensuring better venous drainage and limiting the incidence of venous congestion. It is also easier to harvest the flap with the nerve included. Also, these patients have lost their pulp as part of the injury, so the sensory role of the nerve is questionable. The disadvantage of dividing the nerve is the possibility of a painful neuroma at the base of the finger. In addition, harvesting an artery-only flap results in loss of the sensation over the lateral and dorsal skin on the same side, whereas harvesting the flap with the nerve results in loss of sensation over the medial aspect of the digit as well. Also, sensation to the skin island of this flap is provided by the dorsal branch of the proper digital nerve that arises in the palm and not by the segment of the proper digital nerve that passes through the flap. Karacalar and colleagues reported a static two point discrimination (2-PD) of 4 mm, moving 2-PD of 3 mm, and diminished light touch on Semmes-Weinstein assessment in their case.

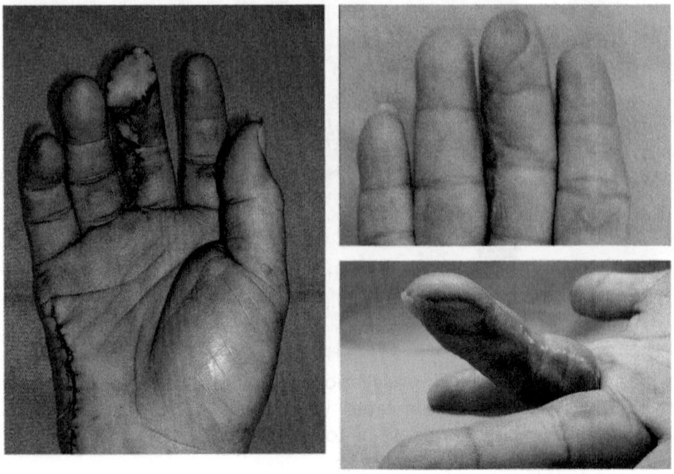

Fig. 6. Use of full-thickness skin graft to cover vascular pedicle in the bridge segment and the flap donor site. Note that the flap has been inset too tightly, making it pale. This was addressed by suture removal and delayed inset with a good outcome at 3 months.

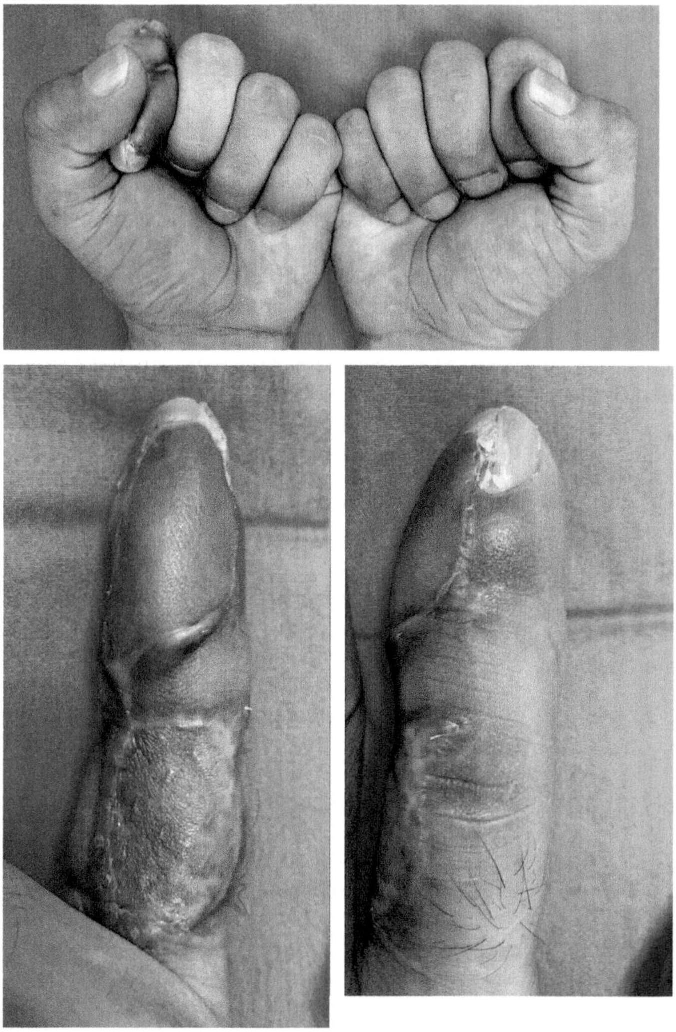

Fig. 7. Outcome at 1 month for patient depicted in **Figs. 1** and **2**.

The cross finger retrograde flow digital artery island flap was described by Lai and colleagues[24] in 1995. In this variation, a retrograde flow digital artery island flap is designed over the proximal phalanx of an adjacent uninjured digit and used to cover the defect on the injured defect like a cross finger flap. The pedicle is divided after 2 to 3 weeks. This variation is useful in patients in whom a standard reverse vascular island flap is not possible because of injury to the digital arteries or the transverse anastomotic arches, and a cross finger flap does not sit well because the defect is predominantly on the dorsolateral aspect. Lai and colleagues suggested the use of this flap to reconstruct soft tissue defects associated with segmental loss of the digital nerve. The disadvantages of this variation include injury to an uninjured finger, sacrifice of the digital artery, the need for a second procedure, and risk of stiffness from immobilization. Lai and colleagues reported 2 patients in whom they used this technique. The flaps were divided at 14 days and 12 days. There was some epidermolysis in the first case, but the flap survived fully. Both flaps had a moving 2-PD of 5 mm at 7 months follow-up.

The heterodigital variation of this flap was described by Adani and colleagues[20] in 1999. In this variation, a dorsolateral flap from the middle phalanx based on the digital artery is raised from the adjacent uninjured finger. The common digital artery, between the injured finger and the donor finger, is ligated and transected just before its bifurcation. The 2 converging branches of the digital arteries are mobilized as a continuous vascular pedicle for the flap. The flap is now vascularized by reverse flow through the proximal transverse anastomotic arch at the level of the C1 pulley. The flap can be made sensate by harvesting the dorsal branch along with the flap and performing a nerve repair. The main indication for this flap is a large pulp defect of the middle finger that extends proximal to the middle transverse anastomotic arch or an associated digital artery injury where it is not possible to perform a standard retrograde flow digital artery flap or a heterodigital antegrade flow vascular island flap. The disadvantages of this flap include the extensive dissection required, injury caused to an uninjured digit, and the sacrifice of a common digital artery. Adani and colleagues reported outcomes of this flap that were used in 6 patients. Five were for pulp reconstruction and 1 was for covering a dorsal digital defect. They had mild venous congestion in 1 case, and the static 2-PD over the flap was between 6 and 15 mm.

DISADVANTAGES

The main disadvantages associated with retrograde flow digital artery flaps include the following:

1. Technically challenging dissection
2. Sacrifice of a digital artery
3. Sensory loss from division of the nerve branches while elevating flap
4. Donor site requiring skin grafting
5. Venous congestion
6. PIPJ flexion contracture
7. Moderately sensible result (static 2-PD ranges from 4 to 9 mm)[25]

OUTCOMES

A summary of the functional outcomes and complications associated with the standard retrograde digital artery flap is summarized in later discussion.

Arterial insufficiency is uncommon with venous congestion posing a more significant problem. In 1 series[21] of 19 patients who had homodigital reverse vascular and neurovascular island flaps, venous congestion was associated with complete necrosis in 2 patients. Partial necrosis was seen in 3 patients, and epidermal necrosis was seen in 3 patients. Moderate congestion was noted in the remaining flaps, in which edema persisted for several months. Meticulous perivascular dissection to preserve the delicate veins should be performed while striving to isolate the digital nerve.

Lai and colleagues[2] reported a series of 11 patients (10 with fingertip defects and one with a volar defect of the middle phalanx) with survival of all flaps. The motion of the involved digit was not limited, but sensation was affected. All flaps had the ability to detect light touch, sharp from dull stimuli, and hot from cold stimuli without sensory reeducation. The mean values of static and moving 2-PD in the flap were 6.5 and 3.5 mm, respectively. Only 33% of the donor sites could obtain measurable static 2-PD of 8 mm. The mean moving 2-PD of the donor site was 5.7 mm.

Kojima and colleagues[9] reported a series of 8 flaps with survival of all patients. Flap congestion owing to compression of the vascular pedicle by the overlying skin was reported in 3 cases. In 1 case involving a pulp defect, moving 2-PD was 10 mm 3 years after surgery, and the sensation was hypoesthetic.

Niranjan and Armstrong[16] reported a series of 25 flaps based on the proper digital artery and its dorsal skin branch, including 5 thumbs with 2 partial flap losses. Nineteen patients were followed up for more than 1 year, of whom 12 had a full range of motion and pain-free digits. The remaining 7 patients had associated bone and/or tendon injuries. Ten patients with fingertip reconstructions demonstrated static 2-PD of 8 mm. All patients were able to detect light touch and showed a moist skin surface.

The series of Yazar and colleagues[25] of 66 patients (70 fingers) with fingertip amputations reported normal monofilament testing results in 64 fingers (91.4%) and diminished light touch in 6 fingers. 2-PD results were normal (<6 mm) in 40 fingers and fair (6–10 mm) in 30 fingers (mean 5.7 mm, range 4–9 mm). Complications included 1 partial flap necrosis, 3 flexion contractures, and 2 neuromas.

In the case report of Endo and colleagues[13] of a left ring finger pulp amputation, the homodigital reverse neurovascular island flap based on the proper digital artery and dorsal digital nerve had a moving 2-PD of 4 mm and appreciated light touch with a Semmes-Weinstein No. 6 monofilament after 10 months. The patient recovered full flexion but had a slight extension lag at the distal interphalangeal joint.

In the series by Lai and colleagues[14] of 3 pulp defects, in whom the homodigital reverse neurovascular island flap based on the proper digital artery, dorsal branch of the proper digital nerve, and superficial sensory nerve branch was used, the static and moving 2-PD were reported to be between 5 and 2 and 3 mm, respectively.

AUTHOR PREFERENCES

In the authors' institution, the retrograde flow digital artery flap is used for the same indication as the cross finger flap, that is, extensive pulp loss or volar unfavorable fingertip amputations. The authors think that the best indication for this flap is pulp loss of the middle and ring fingers because cross finger flap reconstruction for these fingers requires a fair degree of PIPJ flexion. The authors do not harvest the proper digital nerve with the

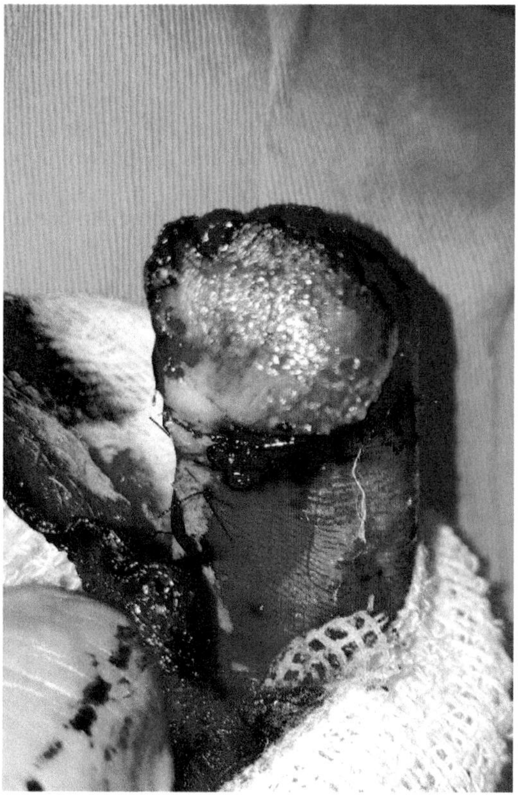

Fig. 8. Venous congestion noted at postoperative day 1. This was managed by suture removal and delayed inset.

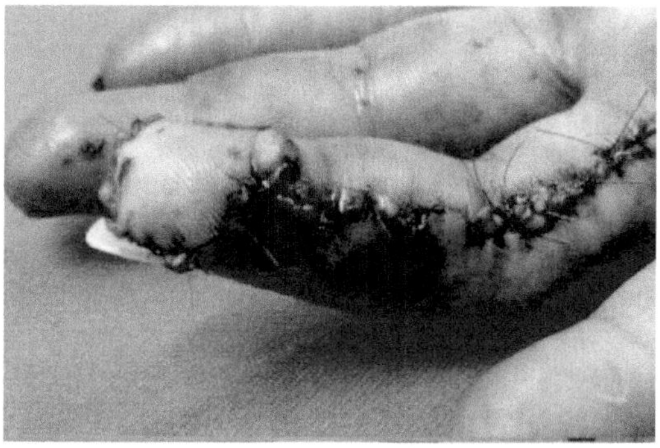

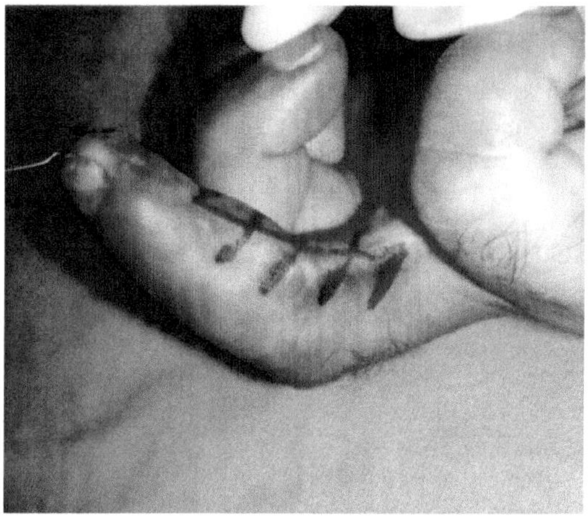

Fig. 10. Linear closure of the flap donor site resulting in a PIPJ flexion contracture. Multiple Z-plasties designed for release of contracture.

flap. The authors' department performed 75 retrograde flow digital artery flaps between 2000 and 2009.[26] They represented approximately 9% of all finger flaps done in their department in that period. Six patients with this flap required reoperation; this included 3 patients with scar contracture, 1 patient each with flap congestion, partial flap loss, and complete flap loss, respectively. The main postoperative complication was venous congestion (**Fig. 8**). Venous congestion can be prevented by suturing the flap loosely and addressed by removing a few sutures especially over the bridge segment and doing a delayed inset after 4 to 5 days (**Fig. 9**). Designing the flap in a "speech balloon" fashion will avoid constricting the skin closure over the vascular pedicle. Scar contracture (**Fig. 10**) at the PIPJ can be avoided

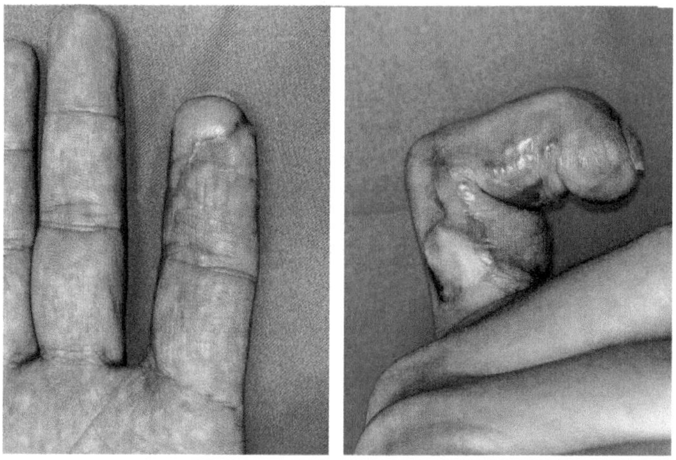

Fig. 9. Outcome at 6 months for patient depicted in **Fig. 8**.

by skin grafting the donor site instead of attempting a tight linear closure.

SUMMARY

The retrograde flow digital artery flap had its origins as a single-stage reconstructive technique for defect coverage from the proximal phalanx to the fingertip. Its subsequent evolution to include neurorrhaphy for sensory restoration made for a valuable addition to any microsurgeon's armament of flaps. Modifications based on branches of the proper digital artery and nerve further opened up possibilities. This article highlighted the technically challenging aspects of flap dissection, described potential complications of flexion contracture formation and venous congestion, and provided technical solutions to addressing and preventing such issues from surfacing.

REFERENCES

1. Weeks PM, Wray RC. Management of acute hand injury. St Louis (MO): Mosby; 1973.
2. Lai CS, Lin SD, Yang CC. The reverse digital artery flap for fingertip reconstruction. Ann Plast Surg 1989;22(6):495–500.
3. Yamamoto H. Anatomisch-Stereoskopische Rotgenuntersuchungen uber die Hand und Fingerarterien der Japaner. Kaibogaku Zasshi 1939;14:837.
4. Saito H. Corrosion anatomical study of the Japanese digital artery. In: Kaibogaku-Kyoshitsu Gyosekishu. 15. Tokyo: Jikei University School of Medicine; 1956. p. 1.
5. Edwards EA. Organization of the small arteries of the hand and digits. Am J Surg 1960;99:837–46.
6. Zbrodowski A, Gajisin S, Grodecki J. The anatomy of the digitopalmar arches. J Bone Joint Surg Br 1981; 63-B(1):108–13.
7. Cormack GC, Lamberty BGH. The arterial anatomy of skin flaps. Edinburgh (Scotland): Churchill Livingstone; 1986.
8. Strauch B, de Moura W. Arterial system of the fingers. J Hand Surg 1990;15A:148–54.
9. Kojima T, Tsuchida Y, Hirasé Y, et al. Reverse vascular pedicle digital island flap. Br J Plast Surg 1990;43(3):290–5.
10. Brunelli F. Lambeau en îlot digital inverse. GEM Winter Meeting. Paris, December, 1987.
11. Oberlin C, Sarcy JJ, Alnot JY. Apport artériel cutané de la main. Application à la réalisation des lambeaux en îlot. Ann Chir Main 1988;7(2):122–5.
12. Brunelli F, Mathoulin C. Présentation d'un nouveau lambeau en îlot homo-digital sensible à contre-courant. Ann Chir Main 1991;10(1):48–53.
13. Endo T, Kojima T, Hirase Y. Vascular anatomy of the finger dorsum and a new idea for coverage of the finger pulp defect that restores sensation. J Hand Surg Am 1992;17(5):927–32.
14. Lai CS, Lin SD, Chou CK, et al. Innervated reverse digital artery flap through bilateral neurorrhaphy for pulp defects. Br J Plast Surg 1993;46(6):483–8.
15. Sapp JW, Allen RJ, Dupin C. A reversed digital artery island flap for the treatment of fingertip injuries. J Hand Surg Am 1993;18(3):528–34.
16. Niranjan NS, Armstrong JR. A homodigital reverse pedicle island flap in soft tissue reconstruction of the finger and the thumb. J Hand Surg Br 1994; 19(2):135–41.
17. Bene MD, Petrolati M, Raimondi P, et al. Reverse dorsal digital island flap. Plast Reconstr Surg 1994;93(3):552–7.
18. Leupin P, Weil J, Büchler U. The dorsal middle phalangeal finger flap. Mid-term results of 43 cases. J Hand Surg Br 1997;22(3):362–71.
19. Germann G, Rütschle S, Kania N, et al. The reverse pedicle heterodigital cross-finger island flap. J Hand Surg Br 1997;22(1):25–9.
20. Adani R, Busa R, Scagni R, et al. The heterodigital reversed flow neurovascular island flap for fingertip injuries. J Hand Surg Br 1999;24(4):431–6.
21. Karacalar A, Sen C, Ozcan M. A modified reversed digital island flap incorporating the proper digital nerve. Ann Plast Surg 2000;45(1):67–70.
22. Chang KP, Wang WH, Lai CS, et al. Refinement of reverse digital arterial flap for finger defects: surgical technique. J Hand Surg Am 2005;30(3):558–61.
23. Li YF, Cui SS. Innervated reverse island flap based on the end dorsal branch of the digital artery: surgical technique. J Hand Surg Am 2005;30(6):1305–9.
24. Lai CS, Lin SD, Tsai CC, et al. Reverse digital artery neurovascular cross-finger flap. J Hand Surg Am 1995;20(3):397–402.
25. Yazar M, Aydın A, Kurt Yazar S, et al. Sensory recovery of the reverse homodigital island flap in fingertip reconstruction: a review of 66 cases. Acta Orthop Traumatol Turc 2010;44(5):345–51.
26. Karjalainen T, Sebastin SJ, Chee KG, et al. Flap related complications requiring secondary surgery in a series of 851 local flaps used for fingertip reconstruction. J Hand Surg Asian Pac Vol 2019;24(1): 24–9.

Flaps Based on Perforators of the Digital Artery

Yu-Te Lin, MD, MS[a,*], Charles Yuen Yung Loh, MBBS, MSc, MS, MRCS[b,c], Cheng-Hung Lin, MD[c]

KEYWORDS

• Perforator flaps • Finger reconstruction • Finger flap • Pedicled flaps • Digital artery perforator • Pulp defect • Free flaps • Dorsal digital artery

KEY POINTS

- Digital artery perforator (DAP) flap is transferred in a propeller fashion for fingertip reconstruction.
- Skin grafting is required for closure of a wider DAP flap donor site or to prevent compression of pedicle.
- Flaps based on the dorsal branches of the proper digital artery, reversed dorsal digital island flap, lateral digital reverse flap, and refined cross finger flap are alternative perforator-based flaps for finger reconstruction.

INTRODUCTION

Perforator flaps refer to an area of skin that can be raised on a supplying vessel that often traverses connective tissue or muscles. These flaps are suitable for small- to moderate-sized defects, can be designed in a freestyle fashion based on the perforating vessel supplying the area, and can be raised as a pedicled or a free flap.[1] When reconstructing finger defects, a like-for-like approach for reconstructing lost tissues is preferred. The glabrous palmar skin of the finger is unique. In addition, the fingertips are sensate, durable, and stable, serving an important prehensile function. The authors traditionally transferred heterodigital island flaps, toe pulp flap, or the medialis pedis flap for fingertip reconstruction to try and restore glabrous tissue. Other methods of fingertip reconstruction using nonglabrous skin include skin grafts, local flaps, pedicled flaps, and free tissue transfer.[2–9]

Perforator flaps of the finger have their source vessel arising from the proper digital artery and are hence termed digital artery perforator (DAP) flaps. The term "DAP" flap was first used by Koshima and colleagues[8] in 2006. It referred to a flap raised on the lateral aspect of a digit based on a perforating vessel arising from the digital artery close to the distal interphalangeal joint (DIPJ). The size and location of this flap made it suitable for fingertip reconstruction. A similar flap based on the dorsal branch of the digital artery at a more proximal location has also been described for fingertip reconstruction. These perforator-based flaps are suitable for small defects. DAP flaps can be raised either as a pedicled flap or as a free flap with supermicrosurgical techniques for vessel anastomosis. This article aims to summarize the available DAP flaps and their usage and provides some technical tips to improve the success of finger reconstruction using DAP flaps. The authors have also suggested modifications to the DAP flap based on the vascular anatomy that can extend the indications for their use.

Disclosure Statement: The authors have nothing to disclose.
[a] Department of Plastic and Reconstructive Surgery, Chang Gung Memorial Hospital, Chang Gung University College of Medicine, 222 Mai-Chin Road, Keelung City 204, Taiwan; [b] St Andrew's Centre for Burns and Plastic Surgery, Broomfield Hospital, Court Road, Broomfield, Chelmsford CM1 7ET, UK; [c] Department of Plastic and Reconstructive Surgery, Chang Gung Memorial Hospital, Linkou Medical Center, No. 5, Fuxing Street, Guishan District, Taoyuan City 333, Taiwan
* Corresponding author.
E-mail address: linutcgmh@gmail.com

Hand Clin 36 (2020) 57–62
https://doi.org/10.1016/j.hcl.2019.08.007

HISTORICAL REVIEW

Several digital flaps that were based on perforating vessels have been described even before the advent of the perforator or angiosome concept. They include the Atasoy VY advancement flap,[10] based on small perforating vessels from the digital artery in the pulp, cross finger flap,[2] based on dorsal perforating branches of the digital artery in the middle phalanx, and the thenar flap,[3,4] based on perforating branches of the superficial palmar branch of the radial artery in the palm.

The observations on the vascular supply of the terminal segments of the finger were described by Flint in 1955.[2] The angiosome concept was elaborated by Taylor and Palmer[3] in 1987, and they demonstrated the area of skin supplied by the individual perforators. They used ink injection studies and noted the abundance of perforators around the interphalangeal joints of fingers. Strauch and de Moura[4] and Endo and colleagues[5] further examined the arterial system and vascular anatomy of the fingers in 1990 and 1992, respectively. Wei and colleagues[1] demonstrated the use of freestyle perforator flaps where fasciocutaneous flaps could be raised on perforating vessels and used for flap reconstruction.

Ogunro[6] described the dorsal transposition flap for oblique thumb amputations in 1983. Although this flap was based on a perforator, it was not until 1997 that Shibu and colleagues[7] islanded the flap and dissected the flap pedicle based on the dorsal arterial branch. This allowed a greater reach of the flap and was named as the dorsal island homodigital flap. Koshima and colleagues[8] in 2006 described the DAP flap for fingertip reconstruction. This flap was based on a branch of digital artery perforating the thin fascia and adipose tissue at the lateral aspect of the fingers close to the DIPJ.[8]

INDICATIONS/CONTRAINDICATION

The indication for DAP flaps in finger reconstruction depends on the location and size of the defect. Small defects that require glabrous skin, such as the pulp or palmar defects, may benefit from a variety of DAP flaps. Fingertip defects can be reconstructed with DAP flaps pedicled and pivoted about the perforating vessel at the level of the DIPJ. Patients with multiple comorbidities who can only tolerate local anesthesia would be better suited for DAP flap reconstruction. It is relatively quicker with a superior outcome compared with skin grafts. Patients who desire a faster return to work, with distal traumatic injuries without the availability of a microscope for free tissue transfer and without the time for a second stage for flap division or delayed procedure, should be considered for a DAP flap.

Contraindications include larger defects that could result in greater donor site morbidity. Fingers with previous surgical scars that may injure the small perforating vessels are a contraindication to DAP flaps. Patients who have vasospastic disorders like Raynaud, are heavy smokers, or have arteriopathy from diabetes and so forth are a relative contraindication with higher rates of flap failure. Also, trauma with a wider zone of soft tissue injury/degloving is also a contraindication to DAP flaps, as perforator damage is suspect.

SURGICAL ANATOMY

The ulnar digital artery is larger than the radial in the thumb, index, and long finger. In the ring and small fingers, the radial digital artery is usually larger.[4] There are 3 major arches in the digits, which communicate between the radial and ulnar digital arteries. The proximal and middle arches are usually found at the level of the C1 and C3 cruciate pulleys, respectively. The distal arch in the finger lies just distal to the insertion of the flexor digitorum profundus and is formed by convergence of the digital arteries in the pulp. The terminal ends of these arteries give rise to 2 to 3 subungual arcades that vascularize the nail bed. The superficial arcade of the nail bed lies most proximal, just dorsal at the level of the DIPJ. It is these vessels that supply the dorsal island homodigital flap in fingertip reconstruction reported by Shibu and colleagues.[7] The digital arteries each have palmar and dorsal perforating branches. There are roughly 4 to 7 branching perforators from the palmar and dorsal side of the digital arteries. Dorsally, the 4 branches have a standard pattern, which corresponds to the condylar vessels, metaphyseal, dorsal skin at the mid phalangeal level, and the transverse palmar arch vessel. The largest of these anastomosing branches occurs in the proximal phalanx, where the dorsal skin vessel and the dorsal branch of the proximal transverse palmar arterial arch are found.

Based on vascular anatomy, various flaps have been described in the literatures. Del Bene and colleagues[11] and Tremolada and colleagues[12] dissected the reversed dorsal digital island flap and the subcutaneous lateral digital reverse flap for finger reconstruction. Based on the perforators of the digital arteries, Beltran and Romero[9] reported a transposition flap from

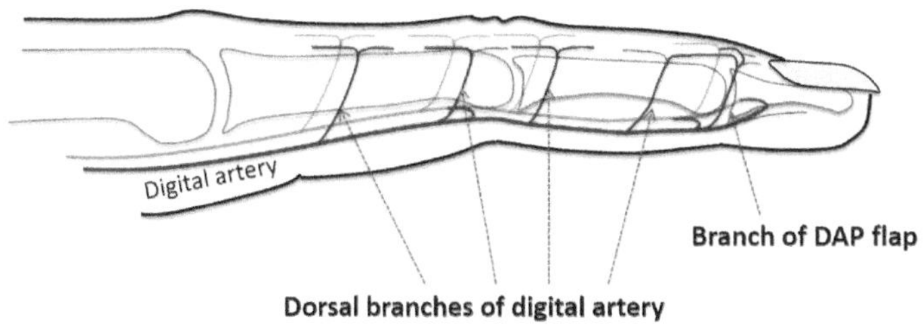

Fig. 1. The location and distribution of perforating branches from the proper digital arteries from which multiple perforator-based flaps have been described.

the lateral proximal phalanx to cover palmar and dorsal defects of fingers. Chen and colleagues[10] reported the largest series of dorsal homodigital island flaps based on the dorsal branch of the digital artery. They selected the nearest uninjured dorsal branches of the digital artery as the vascular pedicle and transferred the flaps from the middle phalanx in 117 fingers and from the proximal phalanx in 70 fingers. This expanded the application of the DAP flaps. They recommended designing the flap 10% to 15% larger than the defect. Chong and colleagues[13] refined the cross finger flap by using the dorsal branches originating from the proper digital artery, dorsal branches originating from the digital arches, and the DAP. The donor site could be closed linearly. For cases with flexion contracture of the proximal interphalangeal joint (PIMJ), the authors raised the adipofascial tissues on lateral surface of the proximal phalanx to cover the defect after stepwise release of the volar plate. The adipofascial flap relies on the same perforating vessels (**Fig. 1**).

OPERATIVE TECHNIQUE/VARIATIONS

A dorsocommissural flap can be raised with the perforating pedicle around the PIPJ. Valenti and colleagues[14] described the flap where the skin paddle was designed around the dorsum of the third, fourth, or fifth metacarpal heads, and a fibroadipose pedicle containing a subdermal plexus was included in the pedicle, which was then pivoted around the PIPJ of the finger to reconstruct distant finger defects.

Fingertip defects have been reconstructed with islanded DAP flaps from the palmar or lateral surface of the finger and rotated 180° and inset to fingertip defects[15,16] (**Fig. 2**). When the skin paddle is taken from the dorsal surface of the finger,[11,18] the flap is dissected from the dorsum to the lateral aspect of the finger. The deep plane at the dorsum is on the surface of extensor paratenon. The flap is raised, and the pedicled soft tissue is dissected toward the lateral surface of the DIPJ, in which the DAP is included. Usually the Grayson and Cleland ligaments are divided to enhance the rotation of the DAP flap. The donor sites are either closed linearly or skin grafted, which may be better on the dorsal surface of the finger.

Tremolada and colleagues[12] in 1998 described a DAP flap based on the distal dorsal branches of the digital artery that could be pedicled on the dorsolateral subcutaneous vascular network. An adipofascial flap is raised proximally and turned over distally to cover defects with a skin graft onto the adipofascial flap. A variety of dorsal turnover transposition flaps pivoted on the anastomoses between the palmar and dorsal vascular network have been described for distal finger defects.[18]

The DAP flap has also been transferred as an innervated flap.[17] The sensory nerve is dissected

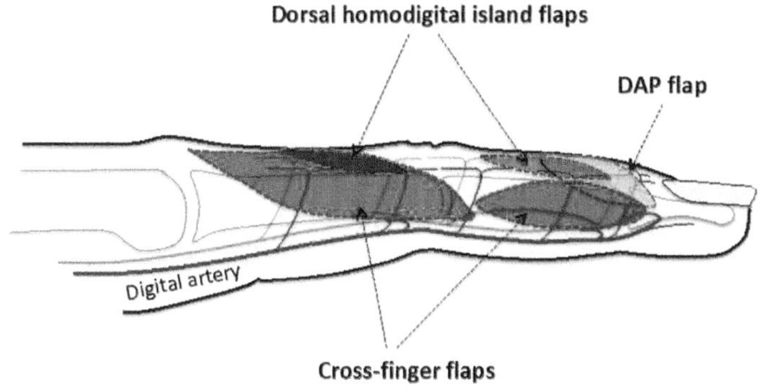

Fig. 2. The cutaneous territory of the DAP flap, dorsal homodigital island flaps, and refined cross finger flaps.

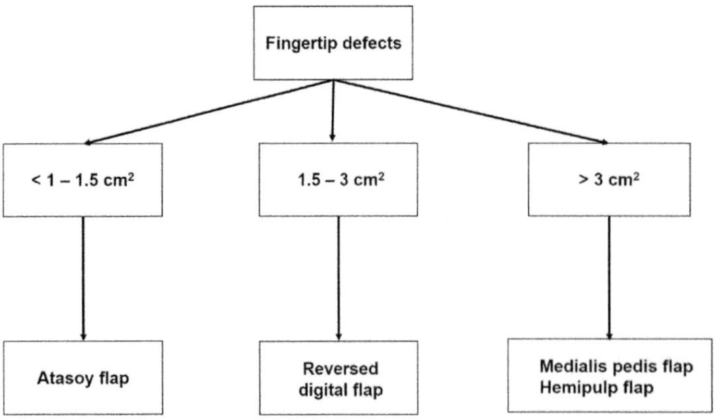

Fig. 3. The authors' algorithm for reconstructing fingertip defects.

from the proximal margin of the flap and is included for transfer. The sensory nerve may originate from the dorsal branch of the digital nerve, the dorsal digital nerve, or the superficial branch of the radial nerve. After inset, the nerve is repaired to the stump of the digital nerve. Two-point discrimination (2-PD) of the flap has been reported to be from 3.4 to 8.1 mm.[19,20] On the other hand, Ozcanli and Cavit[19] reported that there was no significant difference of 2-PD between the DAP with and without reinnervation.

The Boomerang flap, a pedicled dorsal digital artery flap, has been described for reconstructing dorsal distal finger defects. The division of the dorsal metacarpal artery and creating a retrograde flow to the flap from the adjacent finger's dorsal digital artery are the thought processes behind the Boomerang flap. The flap is designed like a Boomerang, with one-half over the adjacent digit and pedicled over the injured digit. When the flap is elevated and the Boomerang is straightened, the flap is able to resurface distal dorsal finger defects.[21,22] The Boomerang flap can also be innervated when the dorsal sensory branches of the proper digital nerve are included in the flap. When transferred to a fingertip defect, where sensation is important, coaptation of these sensory branches to the divided ends of the digital nerves in the pulp can be performed.[23]

The authors also used the DAP-based flap to design the cross finger flap.[13] The modification allows for direct closure of donor site without skin grafting. The flap is not only used for fingertip reconstruction, but also for the defects on volar or dorsal surfaces at different level of the finger. Flap dimension ranged from 13 × 7 mm to 40 × 13 mm. Flap dissection was performed from proximal toward distal finger, and on the surface of extensor paratenon or the periosteum on the lateral finger. It was unnecessary to identify the small perforators. With specific designs, the flap could cover the defects of the fingertip as well as palmar and dorsal finger defects.

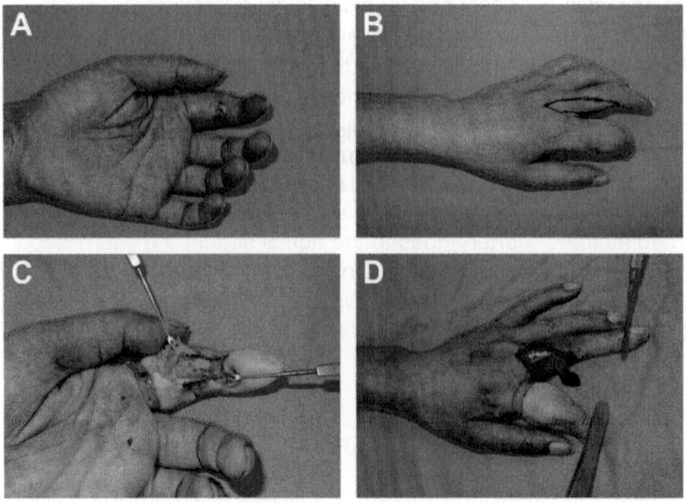

Fig. 4. (*A*) Left index finger PIPJ contracture with a soft tissue defect and inability to fully extend the digit. (*B*) Preoperative marking of the DAP flap on the adjacent finger used in a delayed procedure. (*C*) Release of contracture with the associated soft tissue defect as seen. (*D*) DAP flap raised distal to proximal as seen and perfused by the pedicle around the PIPJ.

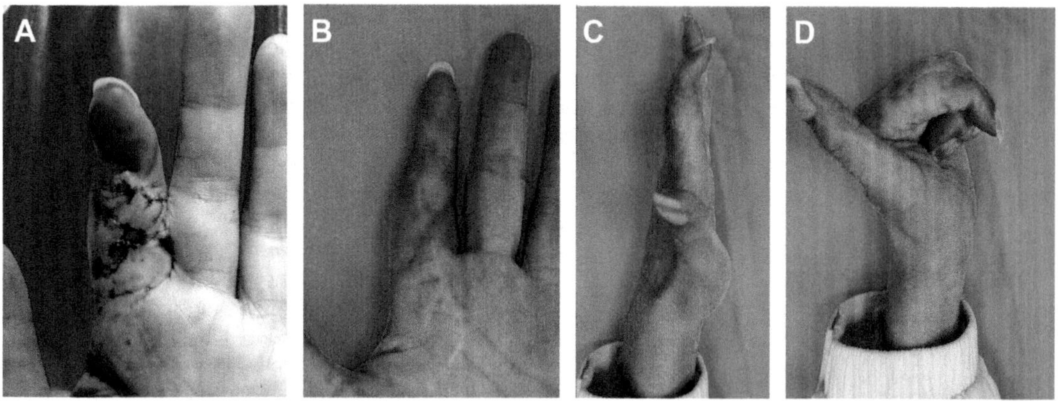

Fig. 5. (*A*) Flap perfused and inset at 3 weeks before division from the middle finger. (*B–D*) Postoperative photographs at 3 months showing the index finger in full extension after soft tissue coverage.

AUTHOR PREFERENCES

The authors' preference would depend on the size of the defect on the fingertip and the resulting donor site defect. Larger defects where donor sites cannot be closed directly are not preferred in the authors' experience. For defects less than 1.5 cm^2, the VY advancement flap described by Atasoy and the DAP flap can be considered. If the defect is between 1.5 and 3 cm^2, a reverse digital artery flap is preferred. The donor site for this flap can frequently be closed directly. With defects larger than 3 cm^2, the authors prefer to use a free medialis pedis flap or the toe hemipulp transfer (**Fig. 3**). The medialis pedis flap provides good glabrous skin with a direct closure of the donor site on a non-weight-bearing area of the foot. Hemipulp flap from the big toe or the lesser toes provides good sensitivity, stability, and durability. DAPs are used selectively where possible but often in the fingertips. The perforating arteries around the DIPJ are not reliable if a more extensive trauma of the finger is encountered. A delayed approach to DAP flap reconstruction may be more reliable in fingers with traumatized or damaged tissues where perfusion may be unreliable (**Figs. 4** and **5**).

OUTCOMES

When the DAP flap uses the perforator close to the DIP joint, the flap is usually transferred in a propeller fashion rather than in an advancement pattern for the fingertip reconstruction. This rotation allows the short-pedicled flap to reach the defect at a distance. Several small case series of DAP flaps have been reported in the literature. The size of the DAP flaps ranged from 2×1 to 4×2 cm^2. The donor site needs a skin graft when a wider flap is harvested. Although none of the series reported flap loss, a potential for venous congestion for the first 4 or 5 days after surgery was mentioned.[17] In the largest series by Chen and colleagues,[10] venous congestion could be observed in 10% of cases, and partial distal flap necrosis could be observed in 8%. Ozcanli and Cavit actually observed even more venous congestion in their series. They suggested avoidance of pedicle kinking.[19]

SUMMARY

Based on the dorsal branch of the digital artery, a flap up to 4×2 cm^2 can be raised to cover defects on the dorsal or palmar aspects of the finger as well as the fingertip. The flap can be safely transferred in a propeller fashion to reach the distal end of the defect. It is important to avoid kinking of the pedicle to reduce complications.

REFERENCES

1. Wei FC, Mardini S. Free-style free flaps. Plast Reconstr Surg 2004;114(4):910–6.
2. Flint MH. Some observation on the vascular supply of the nail bed and terminal segments of the finger. Br J Plast Surg 1955;8:186–95.
3. Taylor GI, Palmer JH. The vascular territories (angiosomes) of the body: experimental study and clinical applications. Br J Plast Surg 1987;40(2):113–41.
4. Strauch B, de Moura W. Arterial system of the fingers. J Hand Surg Am 1990;15(1):148–54.
5. Endo T, Kojima T, Hirase Y. Vascular anatomy of the finger dorsum and a new idea for coverage of the finger pulp defect that restores sensation. J Hand Surg Am 1992;17:927–32.
6. Ogunro O. Dorsal transposition flap for reconstruction of lateral or medial oblique amputations of the thumb with exposure of bone. J Hand Surg 1983;9:894–8.

7. Shibu MM, Tarabe MA, Graham K, et al. Fingertip reconstruction with a dorsal island homodigital flap. Br J Plast Surg 1997;50(2):121–4.
8. Koshima I, Urushibara K, Fukuda N, et al. Digital artery perforator flaps for fingertip reconstructions. Plast Reconstr Surg 2006;118:1579–84.
9. Beltran AG, Romero CJ. The lateral proximal phalanx flap for contractures and soft tissue defects in the proximal interphalangeal joint: an anatomical and clinical study. Hand (N Y) 2017;12:91–7.
10. Chen C, Tang P, Zhang X. The dorsal homodigital island flap based on the dorsal branch of the digital artery: a review of 166 cases. Plast Reconstr Surg 2014;133:519e–29e.
11. Del Bene M, Petrolati M, Raimondi P, et al. Reverse dorsal digital island flap. Plast Reconstr Surg 1994;93(3). 552–537.
12. Tremolada C, Abbiati G, Del Bene M, et al. The subcutaneous laterodigital reverse flap. Plast Reconstr Surg 1998;101(4):1070–4.
13. Chong CW, Lin CH, Lin YT, et al. Refining the cross-finger flap: considerations of flap insetting, aesthetics and donor site morbidity. J Plast Reconstr Aesthet Surg 2018;71:566–72.
14. Valenti P, Masquelet AC, Bégué T. Anatomic basis of a dorso-commissural flap from the 2nd, 3rd and 4th intermetacarpal spaces. Surg Radiol Anat 1990; 12(4):235–9.
15. Mitsunaga N, Mihara M, Koshima I, et al. Digital artery perforator (DAP) flaps: modifications for fingertip and finger stump reconstruction. J Plast Reconstr Aesthet Surg 2010;63(8):1312–7.
16. Kim KS, Yoo SI, Kim DY, et al. Fingertip reconstruction using a volar flap based on the transverse palmar branch of the digital artery. Ann Plast Surg 2001;47(3):263–8.
17. Takeishi M, Shinoda A, Sugiyama A, et al. Innervated reverse dorsal digital island flap for fingertip reconstruction. J Hand Surg Am 2006;31:1094–9.
18. Pelissier P, Casoli V, Bakhach J, et al. Reverse dorsal digital and metacarpal flaps: a review of 27 cases. Plast Reconstr Surg 1999;103(1):159–65.
19. Ozcanli H, Cavit A. Innervated digital artery perforator flap: a versatile technique for fingertip reconstruction. J Hand Surg Am 2015;40:2352–7.
20. Ozcanli H, Coskunfirat OK, Bektas G, et al. Innervated digital artery perforator flap. J Hand Surg Am 2013;38:350–6.
21. Legaillard P, Grangier Y, Casoli V, et al. Le lambeau boomerang: veritable lambeau cross finger pedicule en un temps. Ann Chir Plast Esthet 1996;41:251.
22. Chen SL, Chou TD, Chen SG, et al. The boomerang flap in managing injuries of the dorsum of the distal phalanx. Plast Reconstr Surg 2000;106(4):834–9.
23. Chen SL, Chiou TF. Innervated boomerang flap for finger pulp reconstruction. Injury 2007;38(11): 1273–8.

Flaps Based on Palmar Vessels

Nikhil Panse, MCh, DNB (Plastic Surgery)*, Ameya Bindu, MCh, DNB (Plastic Surgery)[1]

KEYWORDS

• Finger defects • Flaps for finger defects • Palmar flaps for finger defects • Thenar flaps • Hypothenar flaps • Digital reconstruction

KEY POINTS

- Flaps harvested from the palm for digital resurfacing are performed uncommonly. They have precise indications with respect to defect location and dimensions.
- Perforator flaps based on palmar vessels are preferable to reverse flow flaps that sacrifice one of the digital arteries.
- These flaps should be considered for smaller and proximal defects over the palmar aspect of fingers because a secondary defect can be closed linearly.
- Appropriate patient selection, meticulous surgery with delicate tissue handling, and postoperative scar care and physiotherapy help in achieving good results and avoiding complications.

Video content accompanies this article at http://www.hand.theclinics.com.

INTRODUCTION

Posttraumatic and postsurgical skin and soft tissue defects involving palmar aspect of fingers have specific reconstructive needs with regards to the glabrous texture as well as thickness of the skin, color match, and sensibility. In addition to a wide variety of distant or regional flaps, reconstructive hand surgeons now also have intrinsic flaps like homodigital[1–6] or heterodigital[7,8] flaps based on digital vessels at their disposal for soft tissue coverage in complex hand defects. Significant refinements in microsurgical techniques also allow for the use of more sophisticated free tissue transfers using tissues from the foot or toes for sensate reconstruction of defects or entire digits.[9–14]

Sometimes, though, extensive trauma with unavailability of recipient vessels, patient refusal, or lack of infrastructure and skills precludes the use of free-flap coverage. In such cases, alternative means of reconstruction are used.[15,16] Many palmar defects of the fingers are covered with flaps taken from the dorsal aspect of the digits.[2,17–19] The glabrous skin of the palm provides the best color and texture match for reconstruction of palmar aspect of fingers. It follows the principle of reconstructing like with like. However, very few local axial and perforator flaps have been described from the palm for reconstruction of finger defects, the main reason being donor site morbidity. This article is an attempt to review the various local flaps based on palmar vessels for digital reconstruction, and share the authors experience with similar flaps.

HISTORICAL REVIEW

Glicenstein, in 1987, put forth the principle of harvesting flaps based on retrograde blood flow.[20]

Disclosure Statement: The authors have nothing to disclose.
Department of Plastic Surgery, B.J. Govt Medical College, Sassoon Hospital, Pune, Maharashtra, India
[1] Present address: C 902 Welworth Tinseltown, Near LMD Square, Behind Maratha Mandir, Bavdhan, Pune 411021, India.
* Corresponding author. Vimal Niwas, Sudarshan Society, Model Colony, Shivajinagar, Pune 411016, India.
E-mail addresses: nikhil.panse@rediffmail.com; drnikhilpanse@yahoo.co.in

Hand Clin 36 (2020) 63–73
https://doi.org/10.1016/j.hcl.2019.08.006

Since then, Gilbert and Brunelli[21] in 1987, Kojima and colleagues in 1990,[22,23] Zancolli in 1990,[24] Lai and colleagues in 1992,[25] and Brunelli and Mathoulin in 1992[26] have come up with reverse flow flaps on the same principle.

Zancolli[24] described the application of a reverse digital artery island flap taken from the midpalmar area along with the palmar tissue based on the carrier digital vessel, in the *Prensa Midica Argentina.* His technique involved a long islanded flap for coverage of palmar defects of the fingers. The donor site over the palm required skin grafting and was a major drawback of this flap.

This procedure was further modified by Moiemen and Elliot.[20] They thought that their modification, which involved closure of the donor defect by a transverse advancement flaps, produced a more acceptable donor defect in the palm. Apart from these, over the years, few axial pattern flaps were described from the palm for reconstruction of finger defects. A flap based on the superficial palmar branch of the radial artery (SPBRA) has been described and used as a free as well as pedicled flap.[27] Kim and Hwang[28] used the radial midpalmar island flap for reconstructing defects in the first web space. This flap was based on the terminal branch of the superficial palmar arch (SPA).

In an attempt to minimize the morbidity associated with the existing flaps, a greater number of flaps were devised, especially after the concept of perforator flaps was popularized in the 1980s. These flaps had versatile designs and lower morbidity. However, only few perforator-based flaps from the glabrous skin of the palm were described for digital soft tissue reconstruction. Vasconez and colleagues[29] described the use of an arterialized palmar flap, supplied by the cutaneous perforator branches of the index digital artery to resurface the first web. Perforator flaps from the hypothenar eminence were used to resurface the little finger and were especially useful in Dupuytren contracture.[30,31]

Tamer[32] reported the use of a reverse thenar perforator flap harvested from the midpalmar and the thenar region. This flap was based on the dense connections between the SPA, the SPBRA, the princeps pollicis artery, and the deep palmar arch (DPA).

Because of unusual application and donor morbidity, reports of pedicled flap transfers from palm to the fingers and thumb are relatively limited.[22,33–35]

CLINICAL APPLICATIONS

Soft tissue loss of digits needing vascularized cover is always a challenging problem to the reconstructive surgeon. Traditionally, distant random pattern flaps from the trunk, like groin or an abdominal flap, were used to resurface such defects, with their own set of disadvantages, like staged procedure, immobilization, and bulky insensate tissue. Free tissue transfers came into the picture with excellent aesthetic and functional outcomes, but with the need of high technical expertise and infrastructural requirements. Conventional cross finger flaps provide durable and reliable soft tissue coverage, but at the expense of immobilization, multiple surgeries, and an aesthetically unpleasant donor site defect. The ideal flap procedure for resurfacing soft tissue defects of digits should provide a good tissue match with adequate sensations. The donor site deformity should be minimal, with the donor site preferably from the same operative field. It should be a single-stage procedure that does not lead to restricted mobility. Although flaps from the palmar region for resurfacing digital soft tissue defects might fulfill most of these criteria, these flaps are ideal only in a small set of digital defects. They have their own set of advantages and disadvantages, which help in clinical application of these flaps.

Advantages

1. The color, skin thickness, and texture of the flap are well matched to the pulp of the finger and the palmar tissues; so like is replaced by like.
2. These flaps can be reliably made sensate by inclusion of the cutaneous nerve branches and coapting them distally.
3. It is a single-stage procedure without prolonged immobilization, and the donor site of the flap is in the same operative field.
4. The flaps can be customized to the requirement of the defect on the underlying vascular axis in the palm as reverse flow flaps for digital resurfacing.

Disadvantages

1. One of the major axial vessels of the hand is violated. This can lead to finger ischemia and cold intolerance in the affected fingers.
2. Partial sensory deficits and refractory painful neuromas are some of the commonly observed complications.
3. Donor site morbidity with palmar scar contractures results in stiffness, contractures, and loss of functionality. To transfer the tissues from the palm to the fingertips, extensive incisions need to be made in the palm. This resultant scarring over the contact surfaces of the hand can be painful, and postoperative rehabilitation can

be difficult. Most of the drawbacks associated with the use of these flaps, especially those related to the sacrifice of axial digital vessels, can be alleviated by the use of perforator flaps from the palm for digital resurfacing.

The indications, clinical applications, surgical anatomy, and operative techniques of different flaps from palmar tissues are explained in later discussion.

SURGICAL ANATOMY

It is essential to be well versed with the vascular anatomy of the hand as well as its possible variations before executing a palmar flap. The palmar area is supplied primarily by the perforating branches from the SPA and the DPA. These perforating branches have a relatively constant and predictable anatomy, and they form the basis of palmar flaps. Despite many variations, the principal contribution to the SPA is by the ulnar artery, and it is connected to the radial artery by means of various pathways, which have been thoroughly investigated.[36–38]

The SPA lies underneath the palmar aponeurosis and the thenar fascia and is located beyond the distal edge of the transverse carpal ligament. Williams[37] noted that the SPA was formed by the ulnar artery alone in about one-third of patients; in an additional third, it was formed by the ulnar artery with significant contributions from the SPBRA, and in the remaining third, the SPA also has contributions from a branch of the princeps pollicis of thumb or radial digital artery of index finger or, rarely, from the median artery.

The SPA has 3 common palmar digital arteries (the second, third, and fourth common palmar digital arteries [CPDAs]) that course on the surface of the second through to the fourth lumbricals. They run beneath the palmar digital nerve in the proximal region and become superficial to the nerve at a point approximately 25 mm distal to the SPA. The CPDAs divide into 2 proper digital arteries near the metacarpal heads and receive the palmar metacarpal arteries from the DPA.[37]

Omokawa and colleagues[39] have extensively detailed the anastomotic patterns of the palmar vascular arches. They noted that the thenar and midpalmar areas are nourished by perforators that originate in the SPA, the DPA, and the SPBRA.

Vasconez and colleagues[29] demonstrated that the thenar area is nourished by 1 or 2 cutaneous perforators from the radial digital artery of the index finger. Kim and Hwang[28] reported that the supply to the radial aspect of the midpalm is from the cutaneous perforators from the princeps pollicis artery.

According to the vascular anatomy, the midpalmar area can be divided into proximal and distal regions. These regions have different anatomic characteristics. The proximal region has a relatively dense aponeurosis and thin subcutaneous tissue, with smaller and sparsely distributed perforators,[39] whereas the distal midpalmar area has loose aponeurosis with abundant subcutaneous tissue, and a rich vascular supply from the perforators originating from the common and proper digital arteries.[39] Also, the distal thenar and the hypothenar region also has a rich network of cutaneous perforators from the underlying axial vessels and a loose subcutaneous tissue acting as a suitable donor site for the flaps. Thus, the donor areas available for flap harvest are classically located in the inverted pyramid-shaped area of the palm barring the proximal heel of the palm between the thenar and hypothenar region.[39]

In soft tissue resurfacing of the thumb, it is possible to harvest a reverse pedicled radial thenar flap based on the palmar vasculature. Omokawa and colleagues[33] studied in detail the vascular anatomy of the SPBRA in 20 hands. The artery ran just superficial to the tuberosity of the scaphoid and extended distally on the thenar fascia supplying the thenar muscles and overlying skin.

The superficial palmar branch, which communicates with the SPA, was found in a significant number of cases. It is thus anatomically possible to elevate a fasciocutaneous flap from the radial thenar area, using a pedicle created by the retrograde connections of the SPA and the superficial palmar branch.[33]

Further relevant anatomy is discussed in individual flap subsections.

RADIAL THENAR FLAP

Indications

Reverse flow thenar flaps are a suitable alternative to advancement flaps from the thumb or heterodigital flaps for thumb reconstruction. They can also be used as an alternative when free tissue transfer from foot or toes is not an option for various reasons.

Surgical Anatomy

Cutaneous perforators from the SPBRA consistently nourish the skin overlying the thenar area. This skin territory mainly overlies proximal parts of abductor pollicis brevis and opponens pollicis.[40] The superficial palmar branch connects with the SPA in around 60% of cases.[40,41] This vascular connection forms the basis of the reverse flow radial thenar flap.

Operative Technique

Omokawa and colleagues[40] have elaborated the operative technique in great detail. The course of the superficial branch of the radial artery over the thenar eminence is marked with a handheld Doppler. Once the vessel is located by Doppler, flap harvest can be initiated. The authors only harvest the dimensions of flap that are amenable to direct closure so as to avoid graft over the palm. If a larger flap is required, alternative options are considered. After planning in reverse, the flap is marked over the proximal and radial aspect of the thenar eminence overlying the SPBRA. Generally, the flap is planned in such a way that the ulnar margin of the flap is radial to the radial border of the flexor carpi radialis insertion, and the radial border of the flap is ulnar to the superficial branch of the radial nerve and the cephalic vein. The skin and fascia over the thenar eminence are incised, and the inclusion of the artery in the flap is confirmed. Flap harvest thereafter is fairly rapid, taking care not to damage the artery below. The intervening skin between the skin island of the flap and the defect is incised, and the skin flaps are harvested in the subdermal plane so as to keep adequate soft tissue in the pedicle of the flap. A tail like extension can also be planned so as to minimize pressure over the pedicle after rotation and closure of skin flaps. Any thenar muscular branches encountered are ligated. After flap harvest is complete until the pivot point, the tourniquet is released, vascular integrity is confirmed, and flap is transferred to the defect. A clinical series of the radial thenar flap is demonstrated (**Fig. 1**).

Outcome

The radial thenar flap is one of the authors' flaps of choice for reconstruction of the thumb defects. The donor site has an acceptable cosmetic outcome. The authors have not objectively assessed sensory outcomes of these flaps in the long term, but their preliminary experience suggests that they get protective sensations as early as around 6 months. One of the limitations of this flap is the inconsistent vascular anatomy. The vascular pedicle of this flap is not present in all cases, and a preoperative assessment with

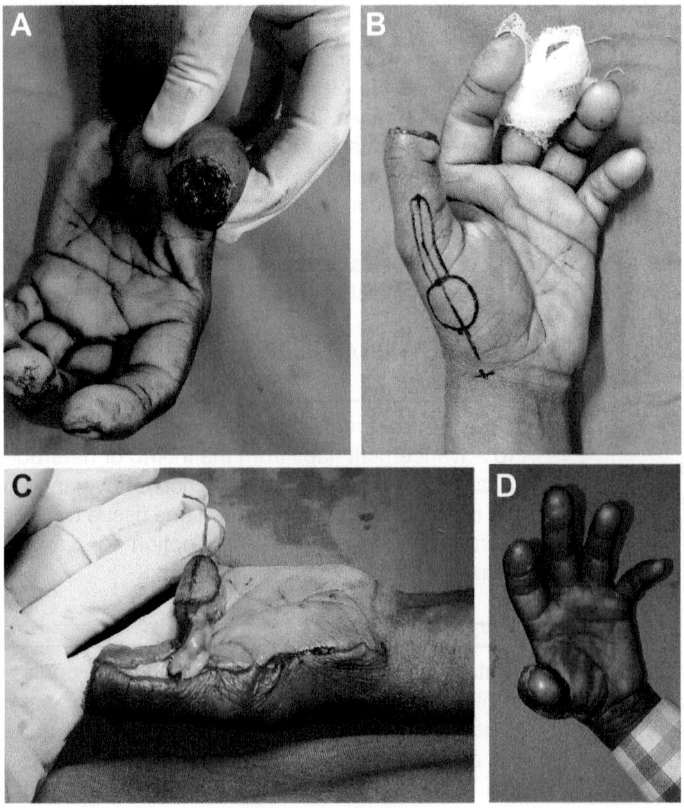

Fig. 1. (*A*) Transverse defect over the thumb. (*B*) Flap markings of the radial thenar flap. (*C*) Harvested flap along with tail until the pivot point with linear closure of donor site. (*D*) Well-settled flap.

Doppler is mandatory before considering this flap as a reconstructive option.

ULNAR HYPOTHENAR FLAP

Indications

A reverse flow–based islanded flap based on the ulnar digital artery of the little finger and harvested from the hypothenar eminence of the hand is a good alternative for reconstruction of palmar skin and soft tissue defects, flexion contractures, or amputation injuries involving the little finger. Especially for palmar soft tissue reconstruction of the little finger, it replaces like with like, and the donor site is closed linearly. In addition, it also has the potential for sensory innervations using the dorsal or palmar cutaneous nerve branches.

Surgical Anatomy

The ulnar digital artery has reliably constant perforator distribution to perfuse the skin overlying the hypothenar eminence.[42]

Three to four perforators are consistently located in the distal half of the hypothenar eminence. The reverse flow palmar hypothenar flap is based on the ulnar digital artery of the little finger. The vascular basis of this flap is from the communications between the radial and ulnar digital arteries of the little finger through dorsal or palmar arterial arcade at the level of proximal interphalangeal joint.[43]

This flap also has the potential of being used as a sensory flap. The branches of the ulnar digital nerve can be coapted to the other digital nerve at the distal phalangeal level.

Operative Technique

The flap is designed on the hypothenar eminence with its axis around the ulnar digital artery. Omokawa and colleagues[42] prefer to take the dorsoulnar incision first to identify and preserve the perforator branches running transversely. The authors now prefer to take the palmar incision first. They think it is much easier and convenient to incise the fascia over the abductor digiti minimi and identify the ulnar digital artery and safeguard its perforators to the skin over the hypothenar eminence. The ulnar digital artery is identified proximally, and the flap is elevated in a subfascial manner, taking care not to damage the pedicle, its perforators, and the soft tissues between the artery and the skin as well as the nerve. The flap is islanded and elevated until the pivot point. The pedicle is not skeletonized, and some amount of fatty tissue is kept near its base. At this point, a vessel clamp is applied to the digital artery proximally; the tourniquet is released, and flap as well as finger perfusion (via the radial digital artery) is confirmed. The ulnar digital artery is then divided proximally, and flap is transferred into the defect. The donor site is closed linearly. A Z-plasty may be incorporated to prevent linear scar contracture.

Outcome

The donor site has an acceptable cosmetic outcome without any significant donor site morbidity. A secondary procedure in the form of multiple Z-plasties may be necessary for the longitudinal scar at the donor site. This flap is not popular mainly because of scarring of the hypothenar area, which might be detrimental to hand function. In addition, sacrifice of the ulnar digital artery to the little finger might lead to vascular insufficiency and ischemia of the finger. The authors have encountered vascular insufficiency of the little fingers despite confirming the presence of the radial digital artery preoperatively by a digital Allen test. With the advent of perforator flaps from the same donor area, the authors do not recommend this flap anymore. Cadaver dissection images demonstrating the harvest and the reach of this flap with important anatomic structures are shown in **Fig. 2**.

MIDPALMAR FLAP

Indications

Midpalmar flaps are not commonly used for resurfacing soft tissue palmar digital defects. They can be considered an alternative to flaps harvested from the dorsal aspect of palm and fingers. When reverse flow homodigital flaps are not a viable option because of compromised vascular arcade proximal to the distal interphalangeal point, the flap harvest site can be shifted more proximally.[23,44–46] The flap can be then based on reverse flow anastomosis in the distal palm or proximal aspect of fingers at the level of proximal phalanx.

Surgical Anatomy

The midpalmar area is supplied by several perforators from the SPA and the common and proper palmar digital arteries.

The terminal branch of SPA forms a confluence with the superficial palmar branch of radial artery or the thumb/index finger vessels, which is located at the junction of the line drawn along the radial border of index finger and the line drawn along the ulnar border of the thumb, which forms the pivot point for these reverse flow flaps.[34]

Two reverse flow flaps from the midpalmar region can be harvested. The first flap design is at

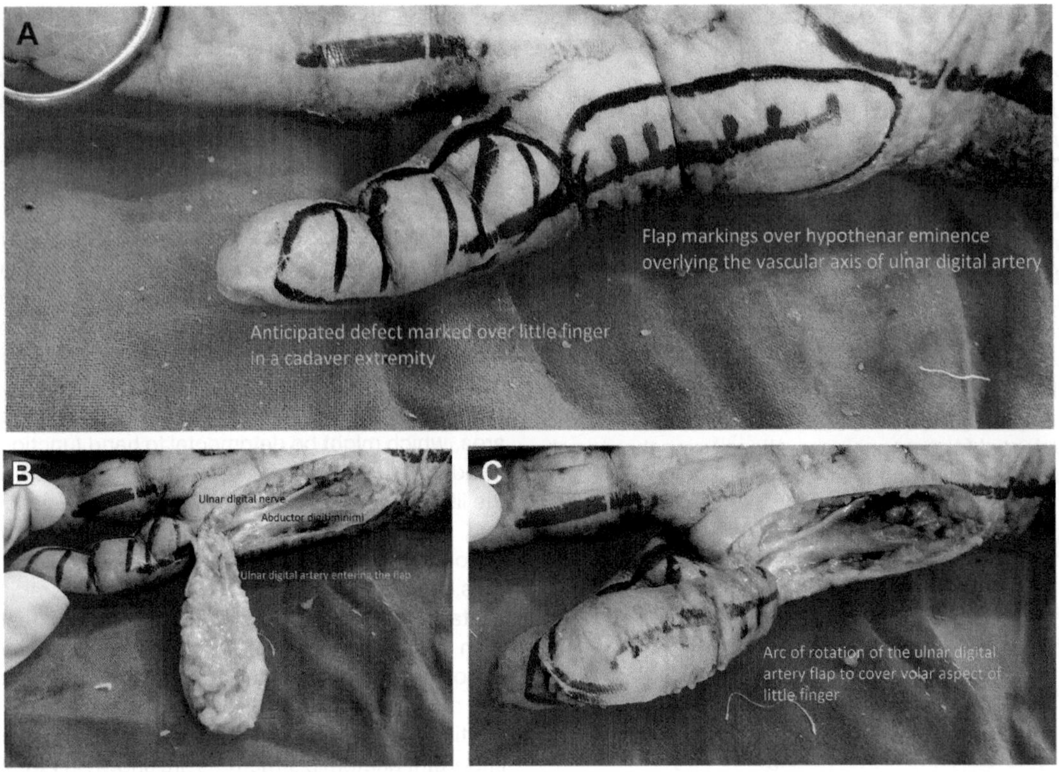

Fig. 2. (*A*) Cadaver flap markings on the hypothenar eminence overlying the vascular arcade. (*B*) Harvested flap with ulnar digital artery entering the flap and the ulnar digital nerve overlying the abductor digiti minimi muscle. (*C*) Arc of rotation of the flap covering entire flexor aspect of the little finger.

the distal midpalmar region based on the reverse flow from the common and proper digital vessels.[24] The second flap that can be harvested from the midpalmar region is from the radial aspect of the midpalm, which is based on the reverse flow through the SPA and its communications with the vessel to index finger or thumb.

Operative Technique

As per the requirement of the defect, planning is done in reverse, and the flap is marked over the palm in longitudinal, oblique, or transverse fashion, so as to facilitate linear closure of the donor site. Flaps are centered on the proper digital artery for midpalmar flaps and over the radial palmar digital artery of index finger for the radial palmar flaps. Flap elevation is initiated from the proximal palm, and it proceeds toward the pivot point. The proximal end of the proper digital artery or the distal end of the common digital artery is ligated, and the flap elevation is continued until the pivot point, including the artery in the flap. Cutaneous perforators of the artery entering the skin are preserved. Utmost care is taken not to damage the digital nerves. Cutaneous nerve branches entering the flap can be included and coapted distally to make it a sensory flap. The pivot point is at the proximal phalangeal level for coverage of fingertip defects or more proximally for proximal defects. Once flap harvest is complete, perfusion of the flap is assessed, and the flap is transferred into the defect. The donor site is closed linearly. Step-by-step harvest in a cadaver hand is demonstrated in **Fig. 3**.

Outcome

These flaps can be considered a viable alternative to the reverse homodigital flaps when the distal arterial connections at the distal phalangeal level are disrupted. However, flap harvest is technically demanding, and the likelihood of nerve injuries is high. Linear closure of the donor sites mandates that the flap width is not more than 1.5 to 2 cm depending on the tissue laxity in that particular patient. The 2-point discrimination for these flaps as evaluated by Omokawa and colleagues[47] in their series of 15 patients was 6 mm in innervated flaps and 10 mm in noninnervated flaps. A proper physiotherapy program ensures full range of motion of the hand and no stiffness at the metacarpophalangeal joint level.

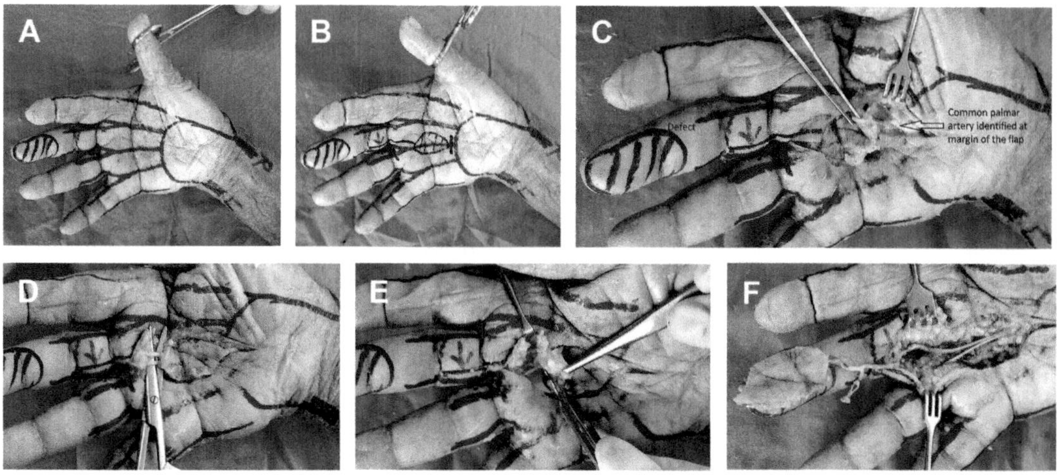

Fig. 3. (*A*) Cadaver surface markings of palmar vessels and defect over the middle fingertip. (*B*) Flap markings overlying the common palmar vessels. (*C*) Common palmar vessel identified at the distal margin of the flap, where it is to be transected and included in the flap. (*D*) Digital nerves identified and safeguarded. (*E*) Bifurcation of the common palmar digital vessel identified. The proper palmar artery going to the ring finger is ligated and transected to move the pivot point upwards, so that the flap can comfortably reach the fingertip. (*F*) Flap reaching the fingertip. The transected and ligated stump of the digital artery to the ring finger can be identified.

Author Preferences

The authors no longer harvest reverse flow flaps from the palm with sacrifice of digital vessels. They prefer perforator flaps from the palm for digital resurfacing, especially when the defects are in the proximal phalangeal area.

PERFORATOR FLAPS FROM PALM FOR DIGITAL RESURFACING

Surgical Anatomy

The distal palm, which has loose aponeurotic tissue and an abundant subcutaneous fat pad, is an area vascularized by perforators arising from the common digital arteries. Omokawa and colleagues[39] encountered that the perforators of this region frequently lie obliquely, and they are more numerous (range, 8–15) with a larger diameter (range, 0.1–0.5 mm) than those of the proximal region, making the distal palmar region more suitable for flap design. The terminal branch of the SPA consistently divides into 3 to 6 cutaneous perforators that supply the radial aspect of the midpalmar area.[39]

Gasiunas and colleagues[48] in their study of palmar perforators of common digital arteries found that 4 to 8 perforators were arising from common digital arteries in the second, third, and fourth intermetacarpal spaces. The average distance between perforator arteries was 6.5 mm, between SPA and proximal perforator artery was 8.2 mm, and between the distal perforator artery and corresponding commissure was 6.3 mm.[48]

Of all the perforators in the distal palm, probably the most studied are the perforators of the ulnar digital artery.[30,49,50]

In the authors' cadaver study, they encountered that there are, on an average, 3 to 4 perforators that are seen arising at regular intervals from the underlying digital artery to form a continuous longitudinal vascular arcade (**Fig. 4**). The consistent and larger perforators lie 3 to 5 mm distal to the distal palmar crease, and flaps can be commonly based on this perforator.[30]

Operative Technique

Most of the perforator flaps that the authors have performed are from the hypothenar eminence for resurfacing of the little finger. After the defect is created, an exploratory incision is made over the palmar aspect of the hypothenar eminence overlying the abductor digiti minimi muscle. The perforators of the ulnar digital artery are visualized. There are, on average, 3 to 4 perforators. The distal-most perforator is visualized about 3 to 5 mm distal to the distal palmar crease. After the perforator is visualized, the distal margin of the flap is committed, and then the flap is elevated and transferred into the defect. A detailed video of the procedure is linked (Video 1). Due care is taken not to damage the ulnar digital artery. Winsauer and colleagues[31] have drawn a line through the pisiform and radial edge of palmar digital crease of the fifth finger and have based their flaps on this axis.

Although the authors have not used these guidelines, they think that it is a good way to

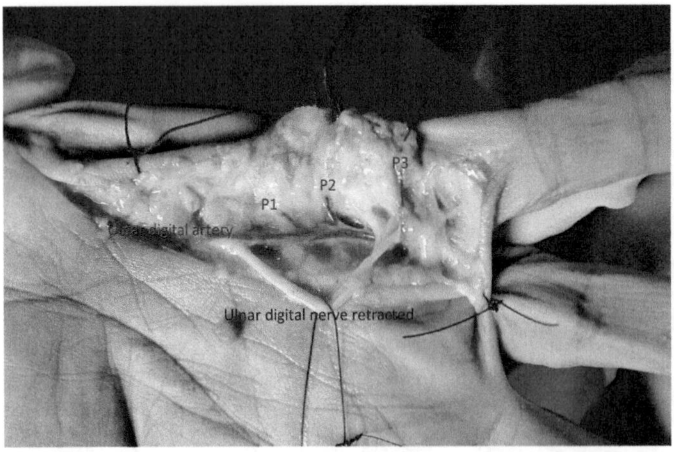

Fig. 4. Dye study demonstrating perforators of the ulnar digital artery (P1, P2 and P3 are the 3 perforating branches).

plan the layout of the flap. In this type of flap harvest, the orientation of the flap is in the longitudinal axis, and the flap is rotated by 180° into the defect. Winsauer and colleagues[31] have noticed a high percentage of partial necrosis in their series. The authors too have noticed a higher incidence of partial necrosis in these flaps. Therefore, they have shifted from a longitudinal to a transverse design. The authors now prefer to design the flaps transversely over the distal palmar crease. The maximum width of the flap is designed to facilitate linear closure of the donor defect. This design requires only up to 90° of flap rotation and permits easier linear closure of the donor site. Similar transversely oriented flaps have been performed by the authors for palmar defects of other fingers. The base of these flaps was just distal to distal palmar crease, and perforators were included in the base of these flaps. Flaps might not be always islanded and can also be performed in a perforator plus manner. The authors prefer these flaps mainly for coverage of defects over the proximal phalanx and middle phalanx region. Clinical series using transverse perforator–based flaps for coverage of defects overlying the proximal phalangeal region for the little finger (**Fig. 5**) and ring finger (**Fig. 6**) are demonstrated. More distal and isolated defects over the fingertips need violation of virgin areas over the proximal or middle phalangeal area, leading to additional scarring over the contact surfaces of the digits and are better avoided. There can also be increased incidence of terminal flap necrosis in such defects. A similar case with distal defect over the index finger was managed by a transversely oriented perforator-based flap from the palm. There was terminal flap necrosis that healed by secondary intention, resulting in contracture of the index finger. The patient was not desirous of further corrective procedures. The donor site healed uneventfully (**Fig. 7**).

The general principles that the authors follow in harvest of palmar flaps are as follows:

1. Damage to the palmar digital arteries must be avoided or else it may result in ischemia of the involved finger.
2. The perforator on which the flap is based is tiny, and spasm owing to traction must be avoided.

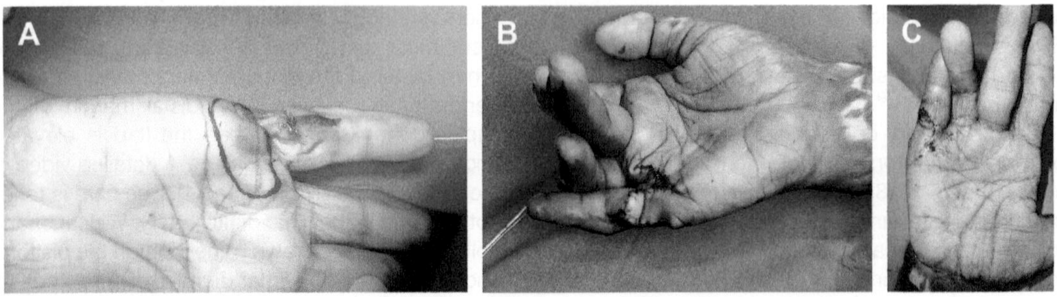

Fig. 5. (*A*) Postburn contracture release defect over the proximal phalangeal area of the little finger and markings of the transversely oriented perforator flap based on perforator of the ulnar digital artery. (*B*) Flap transposed into the defect with linear closure of donor site. (*C*) Well-settled flap.

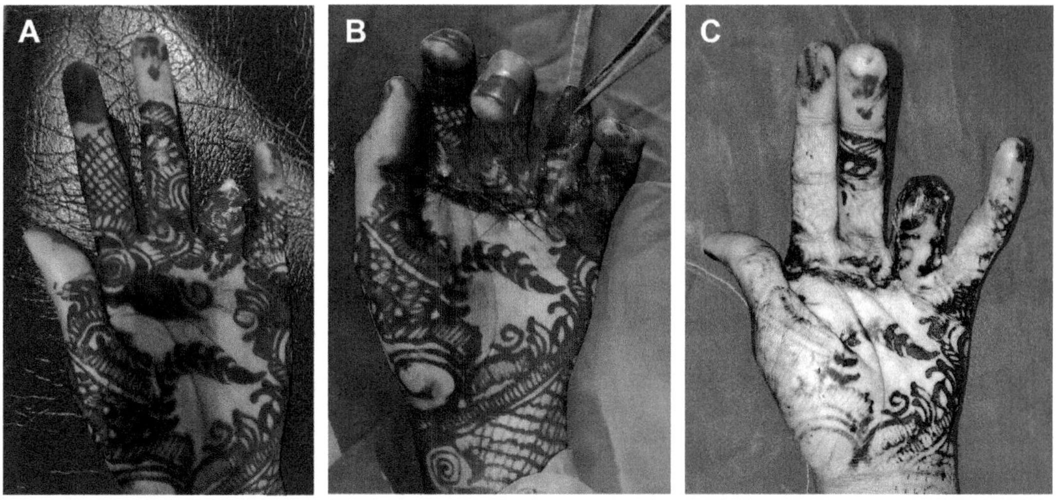

Fig. 6. (*A*) Exposed proximal phalanx of the ring finger owing to trauma. The rest of the hand shows application of henna, which is common during Indian festivals. (*B*) Flap comfortably reaching the defect with donor site being closed linearly. (*C*) Well-settled flap covering the exposed proximal phalanx and the donor site.

3. The perforator must always be kept moist and dilated by bathing it with lignocaine solution.
4. The flap must be permitted to perfuse after tourniquet release before transferring the flap into the defect.
5. The base of the flap must be dissected of all the fibrous strands so as to prevent pressure over the perforator. However, a rim of fat must be left surrounding the perforator.
6. The flap inset must be carried out without tension.

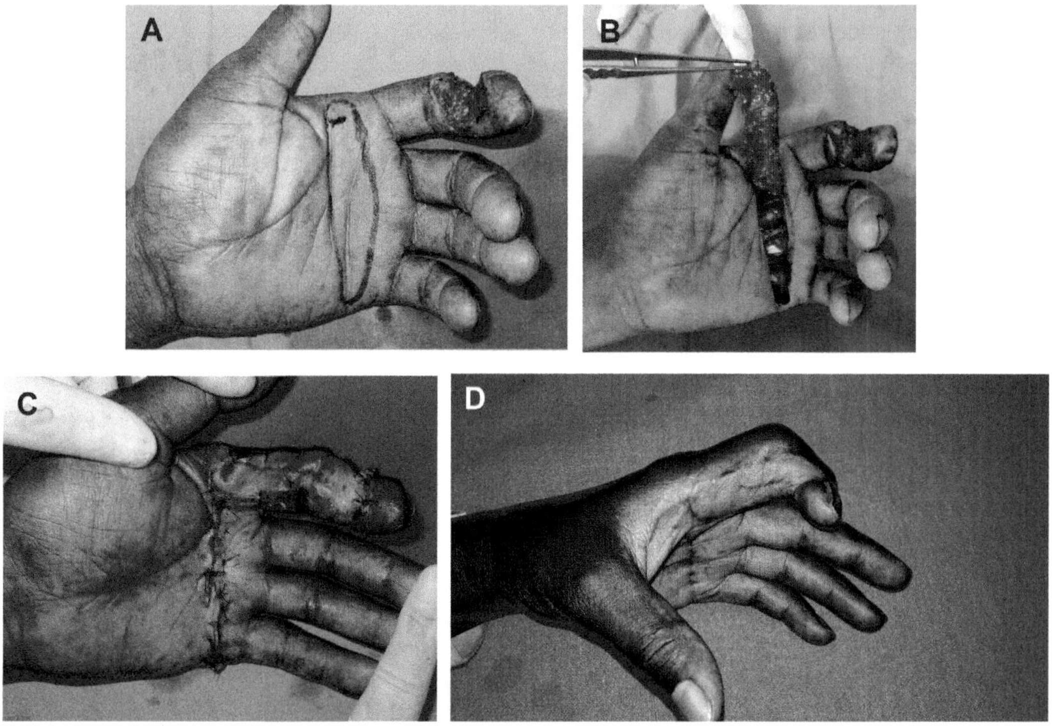

Fig. 7. (*A*) Defect over the index finger with flap markings of the transversely oriented perforator flap from the palm. (*B*) Harvested flap. (*C*) Flap inset over the defect with linear closure of the donor site. (*D*) Terminal necrosis of the flap leading to contracture of the index finger. Also note well-settled donor site scar.

7. Dissection must always be performed under tourniquet control and adequate magnification.
8. Postoperative dressings must be non-compressive.

Outcome

Transversely oriented perforator flaps from the palm for digital soft tissue resurfacing have shown good results. The authors now prefer transverse orientation of these flaps instead of longitudinal orientation. For defects over the proximal and middle phalangeal regions, where linear closure of the donor sites is possible, these are their first choice of flaps.

SUMMARY

Flaps harvested from the palm for digital resurfacing are uncommonly performed flaps. They have very precise indications with respect to defect location and dimensions. The authors suggest use of these flaps for more proximal and smaller digital defects on the palmar aspect of fingers, only when linear closure of donor site is possible. Perforator flaps based on palmar vessels are preferable to reverse flow flaps that sacrifice one of the digital arteries. Appropriate patient selection, meticulous surgery with delicate tissue handling, and postoperative scar care and physiotherapy help in achieving good results and avoiding complications in these flaps.

SUPPLEMENTARY DATA

Supplementary data related to this article can be found online at https://doi.org/10.1016/j.hcl.2019.08.006.

REFERENCES

1. Venkataswami R, Subramanian N. Oblique triangular flap: a new method of repair for oblique amputations of the fingertip and thumb. Plast Reconstr Surg 1980;66:296–300.
2. Hirase Y, Kojima T, Matsuura S. A versatile one-stage neurovascular flap for fingertip reconstruction: the dorsal middle phalangeal finger flap. Plast Reconstr Surg 1992;90:1009.
3. Pelissier P, Casoli V, Bakhach J, et al. Reverse dorsal digital and metacarpal flaps: a review of 27 cases. Plast Reconstr Surg 1999;103:159–65.
4. Foucher G, Smith D, Pemponello C, et al. Homodigital neurovascular island flaps for digital pulp loss. J Hand Surg Br 1989;14:204–8.
5. Henry M, Stutz C. Homodigital antegrade-flow neurovascular pedicle flaps for sensate reconstruction of fingertip amputation injuries. J Hand Surg Am 2006;31:1220–5.
6. Unlu RE, Mengi AS, Kocer U, et al. Dorsal adipofascial turn-over flap for fingertip amputations. J Hand Surg Br 1999;24:525–30.
7. Krag C, Rasmussen KB. The neurovascular island flap for defective sensibility of the thumb. J Bone Joint Surg Br 1975;57:495.
8. Cohen BE, Cronin ED. An innervated cross-finger flap for fingertip reconstruction. Plast Reconstr Surg 1983;72:688.
9. May JW Jr, Chait LA, Cohen BE, et al. Free neurovascular flap from the first web of the foot in hand reconstruction. J Hand Surg Am 1977;2:387.
10. Morrison WA, O'Brien MB, Macleod AM. Thumb reconstruction with a free neurovascular wrap-around flap from the big toe. J Hand Surg Am 1983;5:575.
11. Lee WPA, May JW Jr. Neurosensory free flaps to the hand: indications and donor selection. Hand Clin 1992;8:465.
12. Halbert CF, Wei FC. Neurosensory free flaps. Hand Clin 1997;13:251.
13. Minami A, Usui M, Katoh H, et al. Thumb reconstruction by free sensory flaps from the foot using microsurgical techniques. J Hand Surg 1984;9B:239–44.
14. Koshima I, Etoh H, Moriguchi T andSoeda S. Sixty cases of partial or total toe transfer for repair of finger losses. Plast Reconstr Surg 1993;92:1331–8.
15. Doi K, Hattori S, Kawai S, et al. New procedure on making a thumb: one-stage reconstruction with free neurovascular flap and iliac bone graft. J Hand Surg 1981;6:346–50.
16. Biemer E, Stock W. Total thumb reconstruction: a one-stage reconstruction using an osteo-cutaneous forearm flap. Br J Plast Surg 1983;36:552–65.
17. El-Khatib HA. Clinical experiences with the extended first dorsal metacarpal artery island flap for thumb reconstruction. J Hand Surg 1998;23A:647–52.
18. Germann G, Hornung R, Raff T. Two new applications for the first dorsal metacarpal artery pedicle in the treatment of severe hand injuries. J Hand Surg 1995;20A:525–8.
19. Karacalar A, Ozcan M. A new approach to the reverse dorsal metacarpal artery flap. J Hand Surg 1997;22A:307–10.
20. Moiemen MS, Elliot D. A modification of the Zancolli reverse digital artery flap. J Hand Surg Br 1994;19B:142–6.
21. Gilbert A, Brunelli F. Homodigital island advancement flap. In: Foucher G, editor. Finger and nailbed injuries. Edinburgh (United Kingdom): Churchill Livingstone; 1987. p. 69.
22. Matsuura S, Kojima T, Kinoshita Y, et al. Reverse vascular pedicle thenar island flap. J Plast Reconstruc Surg 1990;10:491–6.

23. Kojima T, Tsuchida Y, Hirase Y, et al. Reverse vascular pedicle digital island flap. Br J Plast Surg 1990;43:290–5.
24. Zancolli EA. Colgajo Cutaneo Isladelhueco de la palma. Prensa Med Argent 1990;77:14.
25. Lai CS, Lin SD, Chou CK, et al. A versatile method for reconstruction of finger defects: reverse digital artery flap. Br J Plast Surg 1992;45(6):443–53.
26. Brunelli F, Mathoulin C. Digital island flaps. In: Gilbert A, Masquelet A, Hertz VR, editors. Pedicle flaps of the upper limb. London: Dunitz; 1992. p. 171–6.
27. Kamei K, Ide Y, Kimura T. A new free thenar flap. Plast Reconstr Surg 1993;92:1380–4.
28. Kim KS, Hwang JH. Radial midpalmar island flap. Plast Reconstr Surg 2005;116:1332–9.
29. Vasconez LO, Velasquez CA, Rumley T. Correction of a first web space contracture with an arterialized palmar flap. In: Gilbert A, Masquelet A, HentzVR, editors. Pedicle flaps of the upper limb. Boston: Little Brown; 1992. p. 135–8.
30. Panse N, Sahasrabudhe P. The ulnar digital artery perforator flap: a new flap for little finger reconstruction, a preliminary report. Indian J Plast Surg 2010; 43(2):190–4.
31. Winsauer S, Gardetto A, Kompatscher P. Pedicled hypothenar perforator flap: indications and clinical application. J Plast Reconstr Aesthet Surg 2016; 69:843–7.
32. Tamer S. Reverse thenar perforator flap for volar hand reconstruction. J Plast Reconstr Aesthet Surg 2009;62:1309–16.
33. Omokawa S, Mizumoto S, Fukui A, et al. Innervated radial thenar flap combined with radial forearm flap transfer for thumb reconstruction. Plast Reconstr Surg 2001;107:152–4.
34. Kojima T, Imai T, Endo T, et al. A study on cutaneous vascularity of the hypothenar region and clinical application as the hypothenar island flap. J Jpn Soc Surg Hand 1988;5:645.
35. Gu YD, Zhang LY, Zhang GM. Hypothenar flap. Chin J Hand Surg 1992;8:865.
36. Botte MJ. Vascular systems. In: Doyle JR, Botte MJ, editors. Surgical anatomy of the hand and upper extremity. 1st edition. Philadelphia: Lippincott Williams & Wilkins; 2003. p. 248–69.
37. Williams PW. Gray's anatomy: the anatomical basis of medicine and surgery. 38th edition. New York: Churchill Livingstone; 1995. p. 1589–91.
38. Tountas CP, Bergman RA. Anatomic variations of the upper extremity. 1st edition. New York: Churchill Livingstone; 1993. p. 187–210.
39. Omokawa S, Tanaka Y, Rhu J, et al. Anatomical consideration of reverse-flow island flap transfers from the midpalm for finger reconstruction. Plast Reconstr Surg 2001;108:2020.
40. Omokawa S, Ryu J, Tang JB, et al. Vascular and neural anatomy of the thenar area of the hand: its surgical applications. Plast Reconstr Surg 1997;99: 116–21.
41. Coleman SS, Anson BJ. Arterial pattern in the hand based upon a study of 650 specimens. Surg Gynecol Obstet 1961;113:409.
42. Omokawa S, Yajima H, Inada Y, et al. A reverse ulnar hypothenar flap for finger reconstruction. Plast Reconstr Surg 2000;106:828–33.
43. Strauch B, De Moura W. Arterial system of the fingers. J Hand Surg Am 1990;15:148.
44. Lai CS, Lin SD, Chou CK, et al. Innervated reverse digital artery flap through bilateral neurorrhaphy for pulp defects. Br J Plast Surg 1993;46:483–8.
45. Li YF, Cui SS. Innervated reverse island flap based on the end dorsal branch of the digital artery: surgical technique. J Hand Surg Am 2005;30:1305–9.
46. Takeishi M, Shinoda A, Sugiyama A, et al. Innervated reverse dorsal digital island flap for fingertip reconstruction. J Hand Surg Am 2006;31:1094–9.
47. Omokawa S, Fujitani R, Dohi Y, et al. Reverse midpalmar island flap transfer for fingertip reconstruction. J Reconstr Microsurg 2009;25:171–80.
48. Gasiunas V, Valbuena S, Valenti P, et al. Volar perforators of common digital arteries: an anatomical study. J Hand Surg Eur Vol 2015;40(3):310–3.
49. Toia F, Marchese M, Boniforti B, et al. The little finger ulnar palmar digital artery perforator flap: anatomical basis. Surg Radiol Anat 2013;35. https://doi.org/10.1007/s00276-013-1091-7.
50. Uchida R, Matsumara H, Imai R, et al. Anatomical study of the perforators from the ulnar palmar digital artery of the little finger and clinical uses of digital artery perforator flaps. Scand J Plast Reconstr Surg Hand Surg 2009;43:90–3.

Flaps Based on the Dorsal Metacarpal Artery

Nicholas Webster, MD, Michel Saint-Cyr, MD*

KEYWORDS

• FDMA • SDMA • Quaba • DMA • Dorsal metacarpal artery • Digital reconstruction

KEY POINTS

- First dorsal metacarpal artery flaps have many modifications to allow them to cover diverse defects of the thumb and index finger. They can be used to restore sensation, venous outflow, and provide durable soft tissue coverage.
- Reverse dorsal metacarpal artery flaps rely on a complex interconnection of the proper palmar digital arteries, palmar metacarpal arteries, and dorsal metacarpal arteries.
- Reverse dorsal metacarpal artery flaps can provide excellent durable coverage of nearly the entire dorsum of each digit.
- The dorsal hand donor site of both reverse and anterograde dorsal metacarpal artery flaps is very forgiving and can either be closed directly or easily skin grafted.

Video content accompanies this article at http://www.hand.theclinics.com.

INTRODUCTION

Flaps based on the dorsal metacarpal arteries are a powerful resource to cover digital defects. They have evolved with the practice of hand surgery over the past 70 years. They can be designed in many ways as simple advancements, transposition, and island flaps. Flaps based on these vessels can provide durable coverage in a single stage for both the palmar and dorsal surfaces of the thumb as well as the proximal palmar and nearly entire dorsal surfaces of the fingers. They are a powerful tool for digital defects that can be modified for numerous situations and have minimal donor morbidity.

HISTORICAL REVIEW

Defects of soft tissue of the digits have been important drivers of development in local flaps to cover these defects. There has been a progressive improvement in the knowledge of vascular anatomy of the hand and potential sources of blood supply to flaps from the hand. Early flaps in the hand and other locations in the body were based on random pattern blood supply and used simple transposition, rotation, and advancement flaps. Simple random pattern flaps are still useful in digital soft tissue reconstruction. But they are limited by the amount of advancement, often requiring 2 stage procedures that can prevent early mobilization.

The development of the neurovascular island flap by Littler in 1946[1] sparked a transition toward island flaps and away from flaps with a cutaneous portion to the pedicle. Island flaps subsequently were developed based on numerous other vessels. In particular, the dorsum of the hand and the dorsal metacarpal arteries were identified as donors. The radial cutaneous branch also provided the possibility of sensory reconstruction.

Hilgenfeldt first described a flap most likely supplied by the first dorsal metacarpal artery in his

Department of Surgery, Division of Plastic Surgery, Baylor Scott and White, 2401 South 31st Street, Temple, TX 76508, USA
* Corresponding author.
E-mail address: michel.saintcyr@bswhealth.org

Hand Clin 36 (2020) 75–83
https://doi.org/10.1016/j.hcl.2019.09.001

book published in 1950.[2] The flap was further developed by Holevich in 1963 as a neurotized racquet flap with branches from the superficial radial nerve.[3,4] Lie and Posch further modified the flap for coverage of the index finger in 1971.[5] All of these flaps likely included the first dorsal metacarpal artery but also included a dermal component to the pedicle. Holevich described elevating an area of epidermis off dermis in association with the first dorsal metacarpal artery creating the handle of the "racquet." In 1979 with a case series and cadaver study Foucher and Braun[6] defined the anatomy for the first dorsal metacarpal artery that the prior flaps were presumably based on and eliminated the dermal component. This created the true island flap and decreased pedicle bulk.

The second dorsal metacarpal artery was described as early as 1928 by Adachi in Japan.[7] Flaps explicitly based on this artery were not published until much later. Lister described a flap likely based on this artery in the 1950s, which he called an axial flag flap from the dorsum of the hand.[8] Earley and Milner performed a cadaver study that confirmed the anatomy of the second dorsal metacarpal artery and helped to outline and popularize the second dorsal metacarpal artery flap.[9,10] They found that the second dorsal metacarpal artery was consistently present and in some cases was larger than the first dorsal metacarpal artery.

Constant distal perforators from the common palmar digital arteries between the metacarpal necks that anastomose with the dorsal metacarpal artery were originally described by Foucher and Braun in 1979.[6] The use of these connections to create flaps based on a retrograde flow was finally described in 1990 by Quaba and Davison[11] as well as Maruyama.[12] Maruyama described a reverse dorsal metacarpal artery flap that included the dorsal metacarpal artery in the dissection requiring dissection of the interosseous muscle fascia and sometimes muscle. Quaba and Davison described the now more frequently performed flap that relies on the recurrent dorsal cutaneous branch of the dorsal metacarpal artery rather than including the entire vessel with the dissection. Quaba and Davison also described harvesting vascularized tendon with their flap. Previous anatomic studies showed that the ulnar dorsal metacarpal arteries become less reliable in their proximal anatomy. This meant third and fourth dorsal metacarpal artery flaps were often not possible. However, the distal perforators of the third and fourth dorsal metacarpal arteries as well as the first and second are consistently present allowing these perforator-based flaps to be raised reliably. This meant a new ability to provide durable soft tissue coverage for the proximal portion of each digit and web space. This greatly improved the versatility of this group of flaps.

In 1997 Karacalar and Özcan showed that the perforating branch from the common palmar metacarpal artery could be ligated. This meant that the flap could be taken based on the terminal branches of the dorsal metacarpal artery that connect to the proper palmar digital arteries. This allowed the pivot point for the flap to move distally to the base of the proximal phalanx. Yang and Morris confirmed this with their anatomic study in 2001.[13]

In 1997 Santa-Comba and colleagues[14] described harvesting the reverse dorsal metacarpal artery flap as an osteocutaneous flap. Proximal phalangeal defects with missing soft tissue, extensor tendon, and bone could now be reconstructed with a single flap.

There are numerous variants of dorsal metacarpal artery flaps that have been developed. The knowledge of dorsal hand anatomy and the connections between the volar and dorsal hand have resulted in new homodigital flaps and further refinement of digital reconstruction with local flaps.

INDICATIONS/CONTRAINDICATIONS

First Dorsal Metacarpal Artery Flaps

The first dorsal metacarpal artery flap is known for its use in reconstruction of the soft tissue of the thumb. It can in its various forms reconstruct nearly the entire dorsum or palmar surface of the thumb. It is also useful in first web space contractures (**Fig. 1**).

Second Dorsal Metacarpal Artery Flaps

The second dorsal metacarpal artery flap is indicated to cover thumb defects, the palmar proximal index and long fingers, and nearly the entire dorsum of either the index or the long finger (**Figs. 2** and **3**).

Third and Fourth Dorsal Metacarpal Artery Flaps

These flaps can be designed to cover similar type defects to the second dorsal metacarpal artery flaps. They are almost entirely designed as reverse flaps due to the less consistent anatomy in the third and fourth dorsal metacarpal arteries. **Fig. 2** illustrates the small size of these arteries relative to the first and second in the proximal hand.

CONTRAINDICATIONS

All dorsal metacarpal artery flaps are contraindicated if there is prior surgery that may have

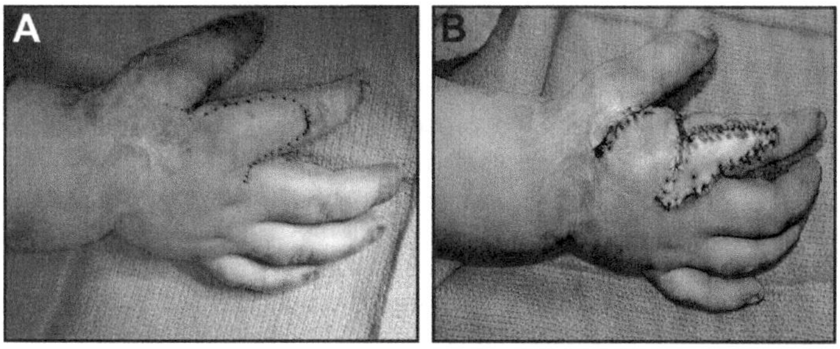

Fig. 1. (*A, B*) An example of first web space reconstruction for a burn contracture in a young child. As all vascularized tissues, it is best used when there is a need for durable coverage over tendon, bone, or neurovascular structures. The first dorsal metacarpal artery flap can also be modified to cover defects of the palmar and dorsal proximal index finger. It can be used in replants to reconstruct dorsal veins as a venous flow through flap.

divided the perforating vessels or dorsal metacarpal artery that supplies these flaps. Use caution when designing flaps that have scars crossing them. The dorsal hand frequently has sun damaged skin that can contain undiagnosed skin cancers. Pay close attention to any skin lesion that might be transposed to the finger.

SURGICAL ANATOMY

The proximal dorsal hand is supplied by the dorsal metacarpal arch through the dorsal metacarpal arteries. The distal dorsal hand and dorsal area of the proximal phalanx are supplied by perforators of the deep palmar arch.[13] These 2 systems are interconnected allowing for retrograde flaps.

The first dorsal metacarpal artery originates from the radial artery just distal to the extensor pollicis longus tendon. The first dorsal metacarpal artery was shown in cadaver dissections by Sherif[15] to have 3 relatively constant branches. The most important branch is described as the ulnar branch. This branch travels along the radial dorsal border of the second metacarpal just superficial to the deep interosseous muscle fascia deep to the extensor tendons. The ulnar branch is deep to the fascia and within the interosseous muscle 15% of the time according to the series of dissections by Earley[9] but is always superficial at the distal extent near the metacarpal neck. The radial branch runs along the dorsum of the first metacarpal. The remaining intermediate branch travels through the center of the first web space. The ulnar, radial, and intermediate branches of the first dorsal metacarpal artery anastomose with one another and perforators from the palmar hand distally. The ulnar branch in 70% of cases is of significant size, with the intermediate and radial being substantial in about 30% of hands.

The second, third, and fourth dorsal metacarpal arteries generally arise from the dorsal metacarpal arch. Rarely, the second dorsal metacarpal artery may arise directly from the radial artery and the third and fourth dorsal metacarpal arteries may arise from the ulnar artery. The second dorsal metacarpal artery is the most consistent vessel after the first and can occasionally be larger than the first. The arteries run adjacent to the metacarpals within the intermetacarpal space over the

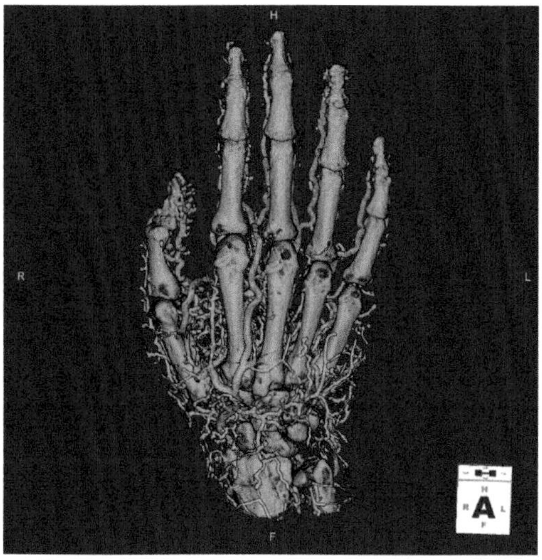

Fig. 2. The large second dorsal metacarpal artery.

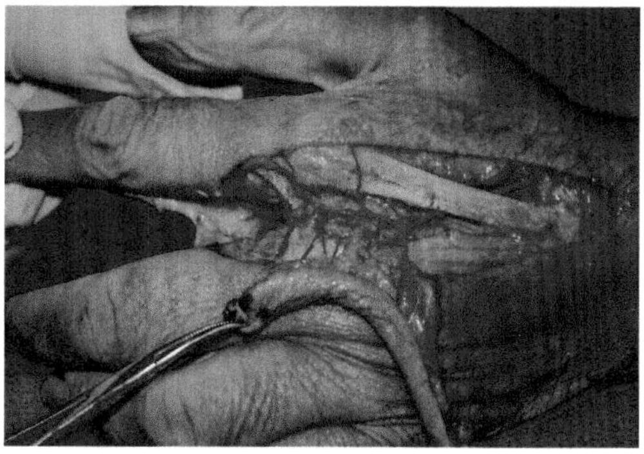

Fig. 3. The numerous small branches to skin from the second dorsal metacarpal artery that provide the robust blood supply to the second web space and dorsal index/long fingers.

interosseous muscle fascia deep to the extensor tendons. They may run deep to the fascia or within the interosseous muscle as the first dorsal metacarpal artery.[10,13]

The first dorsal metacarpal artery and the other dorsal metacarpal arteries all anastomose with adjacent vascular territories. Proximally in the hand they have branches between the dorsal metacarpal arteries. More distally, the dorsal metacarpal arteries join with perforating branches from the deep palmar arch with 1 to 2 perforators per metacarpal space. These perforators are consistently at the level of the metacarpal neck. The most distal extent of the dorsal metacarpal arteries joins with the dorsal cutaneous branches of the palmar digital arteries. Branches of the deep metacarpal artery perforators also join with the branches of the palmar digital arteries. This robust collateral flow allows for the reverse flow flaps[11–13,16] (**Fig. 4**).

OPERATIVE TECHNIQUE/VARIATIONS

The defect is measured, and the required size of the flap is anticipated and transposed. Considerations for design of all dorsal metacarpal artery flaps include coverage of the donor site. The medial arm is frequently a good site of full-thickness skin graft with adequate color match. Reverse flaps often can be closed directly. A pinch test should be performed to confirm this.

First Dorsal Metacarpal Artery Flap

The first dorsal metacarpal artery flap is a workhorse flap for coverage of the thumb. The anterograde first dorsal metacarpal artery flap can be harvested as a true island flap or racquet shaped with a cutaneous tail. It is designed over the dorsum of the index finger proximal phalanx from one midaxial line to the other. The distal extent is traditionally the proximal interphalangeal joint (PIP). The proximal extent in an island flap is the metacarpal phalangeal joint. Once the flap is outlined, a lazy "S" type incision is designed from the head of the second metacarpal to the base of the first web space.

The lazy S access incision is incised, and the first dorsal metacarpal artery is identified near its origin just distal to the extensor pollicis longus. Branches of the radial sensory nerve can be identified that are traveling toward the flap and preserved. One or two dorsal veins are included in the flap to preserve venous outflow. The veins, the first dorsal metacarpal artery, and any included cutaneous nerves are then dissected proximally to distally. The artery will be dissected subfascially but in most cases is suprafascial. In some cases, the artery will dive intramuscularly and will have to be dissected free and branches divided.

Once the pedicle has been freed distally to the skin paddle, the radial aspect of the flap is elevated just superficial to paratenon. It is critical that the flap not be thinned to ensure adequate blood supply. The known perforating branches from the proper palmar digital arteries and the palmar metacarpal arteries can be divided. The flap can then be transposed to cover any defect. The lazy s incision is closed, and a full-thickness skin graft is used to close the donor site.

Modifications of the first dorsal metacarpal artery flap

Extended first dorsal metacarpal artery flap Flaps can be harvested distal to the PIP. The extension beyond the PIP is thought to be based on a random pattern blood supply.[17,18] The first dorsal metacarpal artery can also be harvested including the second dorsal metacarpal artery to provide a large bilobed flap. The entire second web space can be harvested to provide more skin to resurface large thumb defects or first web space defects.[19]

Sensory first dorsal metacarpal artery flap As with the original description of this flap, the branches of the radial nerve can be included to provide sensation. Cortical remodeling is often challenging and incomplete, especially in adults. Alternatively, the radial sensory nerve can be divided and sutured to the proximal stump of the injured digital nerve[20] (**Fig. 5**).

Flow through flap The first dorsal metacarpal artery flap can be used to cover defects of the dorsal thumb during replantation. The dorsal veins that are included in the flap can be divided and used as interposition vein grafts. This can augment venous return in replantation cases. It saves the step of harvesting separate vein grafts in addition

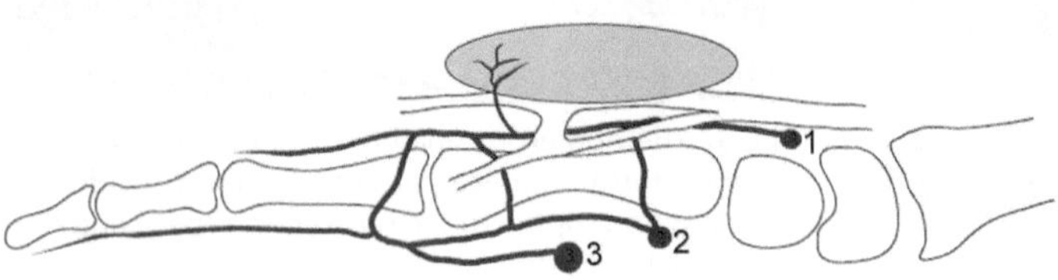

Fig. 4. (1) The dorsal metacarpal arch (2) to the deep palmar arch and (3) the superficial palmar arch.

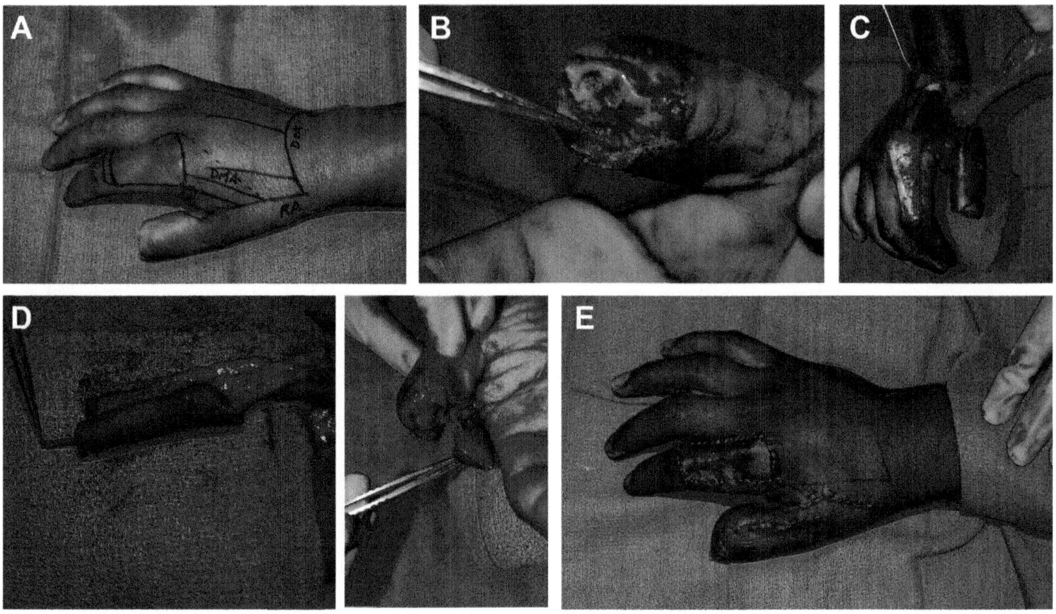

Fig. 5. (*A–E*) Divided radial sensory nerve sutured to the proximal stump of the injured digital nerve.

to a flap to cover the dorsal thumb in these circumstances.[21]

Intact base This flap includes the skin of the dorsal first web space and proximal phalanx. The base is left intact and allows resurfacing the thumb metacarpal as well as the first web space. This decreases the risk of venous congestion and tight closure with tunneled flaps (**Fig. 6**).

Second Dorsal Metacarpal Artery Flap

The second dorsal metacarpal artery flap is very similar to the first dorsal metacarpal artery flap in its applications. It has a wide arc of rotation. It can cover thumb defects but can be used on the adjacent digits. The anterograde flap can be harvested with similar modifications as the first dorsal metacarpal artery flap. The second dorsal metacarpal artery is very consistent in its anatomy.

The second dorsal metacarpal artery through its connections with the proper palmar digital artery perforators supplies the second web space and the ulnar aspect of the dorsal index and the radial aspect of the dorsal long finger. This allows the flap to be designed to include the skin of the dorsal proximal index and or long finger. The flap can also include the skin of the second web space.

The skin paddle is designed. Then a longitudinal access incision is designed over the second intermetacarpal space to the level of the separation of the index and long finger extensor tendons. This is the pivot point for the pedicle of the flap and limits its mobility. The access incision is incised, and the skin elevated leaving dorsal veins intact identifying at least one to include with the pedicle to provide venous outflow for the flap.

The flap is then elevated distal to proximal with care to include all the soft tissue superficial to the paratenon over the metacarpal heads. It is critical to include this soft tissue to prevent vascular embarrassment of the flap. The perforating branches from the palmar metacarpal arteries are divided and the pedicle is identified and elevated subfascially to avoid damage to the artery. As with the first dorsal metacarpal artery flap, it may have a partially submuscular course and may require intramuscular dissection with division of branches to the interosseous muscles.

The flap can then be transposed to cover the defect. The access incision is closed, and a full-thickness skin graft is used to close the donor site.

Modifications of the second dorsal metacarpal artery flap

Extended second dorsal metacarpal artery flap The second dorsal metacarpal artery flap can include harvest of the second web space and the dorsum of the index and long fingers. As the first dorsal metacarpal artery, extended second dorsal metacarpal artery flap distal to the PIP can be harvested on a random pattern basis.[22]

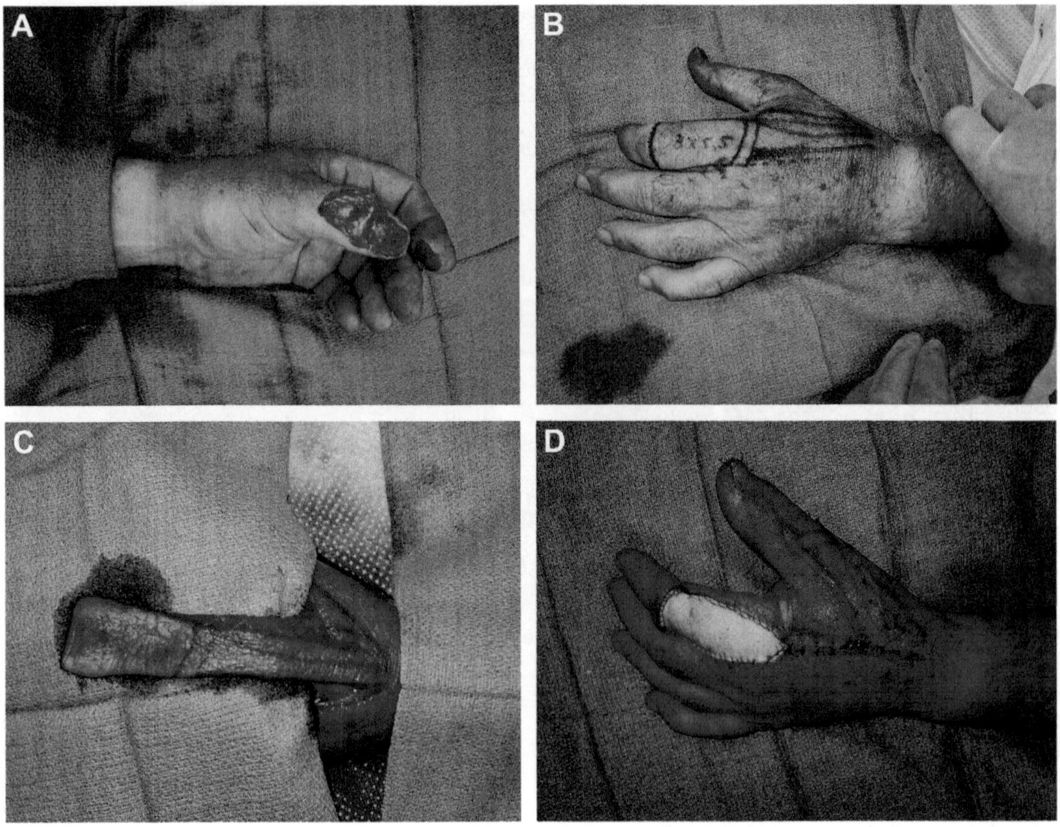

Fig. 6. (*A–D*) Intact base technique on a dorsal thumb defect.

Sensory second dorsal metacarpal artery flap Branches of the radial sensory nerve can be included, especially if the dorsal index skin is being included in the flap. These can be dissected as described earlier but can tether the flap because they have a different pivot point than the second dorsal metacarpal artery flap.

Reverse flow flaps This class of flaps is extremely versatile. They often allow linear closure of their donor site and can cover a diverse group of defects of the dorsal digits and web spaces. They are based on the distal connections between the palmar metacarpal arteries and the dorsal metacarpal arteries and/or the proper palmar digital arteries. Because of the consistency of the connection between the distal dorsal metacarpal arteries and the palmar metacarpal arteries, they can be designed over the second, third, and fourth intermetacarpal spaces based on the second, third, and fourth dorsal metacarpal arteries, respectively. The flap may extend from the metacarpophalangeal joint to the distal wrist crease and vary in width from 1 to 3.5 cm. The pivot point of the flap is generally 0.5 to 1 cm proximal to the adjacent metacarpophalangeal joint.

Once the skin paddle has been designed, the flap is incised on one side down to paratenon. The flap is then elevated proximal to distal. Care is taken distal to the intertendinous connection

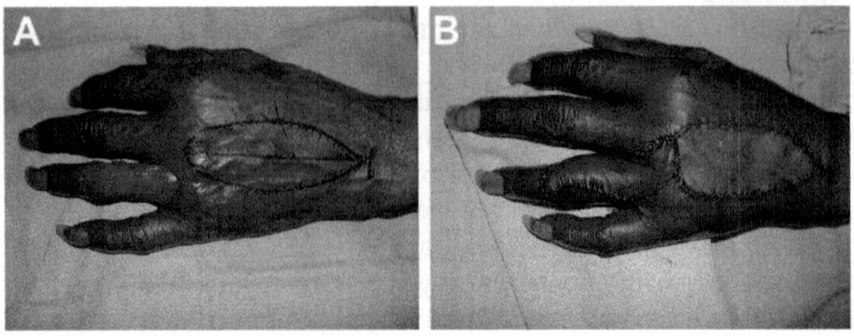

Fig. 7. (*A, B*) A case of loss of a very large portion of the skin of the dorsal index due to a cancer, reconstructed with a large skin paddle.

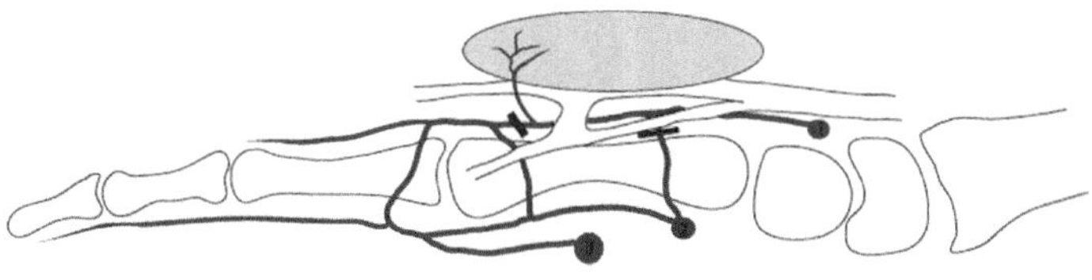

Fig. 8. Development of double pivot dorsal metacarpal artery flap. The black bars represent division of the vessels.

where the perforating branch that supplied the flap is located. Once the pedicle has been identified, the flap incisions are completed and the flap is rotated up to 180° and inset. Do not skeletonize the pedicle, as this may cause kinking or diminish venous outflow.

The donor site can generally be closed linearly, but if there is excessive tension, skin grafting or local flaps can be used to close the donor site. See Video 1 for a video exemplifying the elevation of a reverse dorsal metacarpal artery flap (**Fig. 7**).

Modifications of reverse flow flaps

Double pivot second dorsal metacarpal artery flap This flap is actually an anterograde flow flap but uses the skin paddle design of a reverse flow flap. The flap is elevated in standard reverse flow fashion. The dorsal metacarpal artery is then ligated distal to the recurrent cutaneous perforator branch. The dorsal metacarpal artery is then dissected proximally as a traditional anterograde flap. This allows the skin paddle to rotate 180° as a reverse flow flap. Reverse flow flaps often have better donor site because they take skin from the dorsum of the hand rather than the dorsal proximal finger. This allows for direct closure rather than needing a skin graft. The pivot point for this flap is at the intersection of the index and long fingers in the proximal dorsal hand rather than the metacarpal neck of a tradition reverse flow flap[23] (**Fig. 8**).

Proper digital artery retrograde flow A dorsal metacarpal artery flap can be harvested based on the connections between the recurrent dorsal branch of the dorsal metacarpal artery and the proper digital arteries. The flap is harvested as described earlier but once isolated on the recurrent dorsal branch the dissection is carried deep into the interosseous muscle. The dorsal metacarpal artery is identified distally and proximally to the branch to perforator from the metacarpal artery. This perforator is then divided and the dorsal metacarpal artery proximal to the cutaneous branch is divided as well. This leaves the recurrent dorsal branch connected to the distal dorsal metacarpal artery that connects to the proper digital artery distally. This moves the pivot point of the flap from the distal metacarpal to the proximal phalanx[16] (**Fig. 9**).

Osteocutaneous flap An osteocutaneous flap can be designed to reconstruct bony defects of the proximal phalanx. This can be performed by including the dorsal metacarpal artery in the flap design as described by Maruyama.[12] Proximally the dorsal metacarpal artery is left attached to the fascia and periosteum of the metacarpal.[14] Osteotomies are performed and a small portion of cortical bone can then be transposed distally (**Fig. 10**).

AUTHOR PREFERENCES

First Dorsal Metacarpal Artery Flap

The senior author prefers to design first dorsal metacarpal artery flaps with an intact cutaneous base. This augments venous outflow and prevents the pedicle from being crushed within a tight subcutaneous tunnel. The intervening skin of the first webspace that is, left when transposing this flap for thumb reconstruction is well vascularized by perforating branches from the palmar hand to the intermediate branch of the first dorsal metacarpal artery.

Reverse Flap Modification

Often the distal recurrent cutaneous branch of the dorsal metacarpal artery is not clearly visible, or it can be damaged in dissection. In the authors' experience, the flap can be raised on a broad base of adipofascial tissue distally with division of this branch. This allows the pivot point to

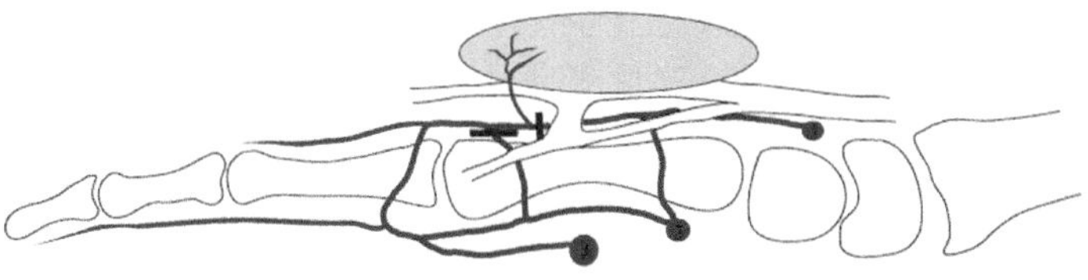

Fig. 9. Development of proper digital artery retrograde flow dorsal metacarpal artery flap. The black bars represent division of the vessels.

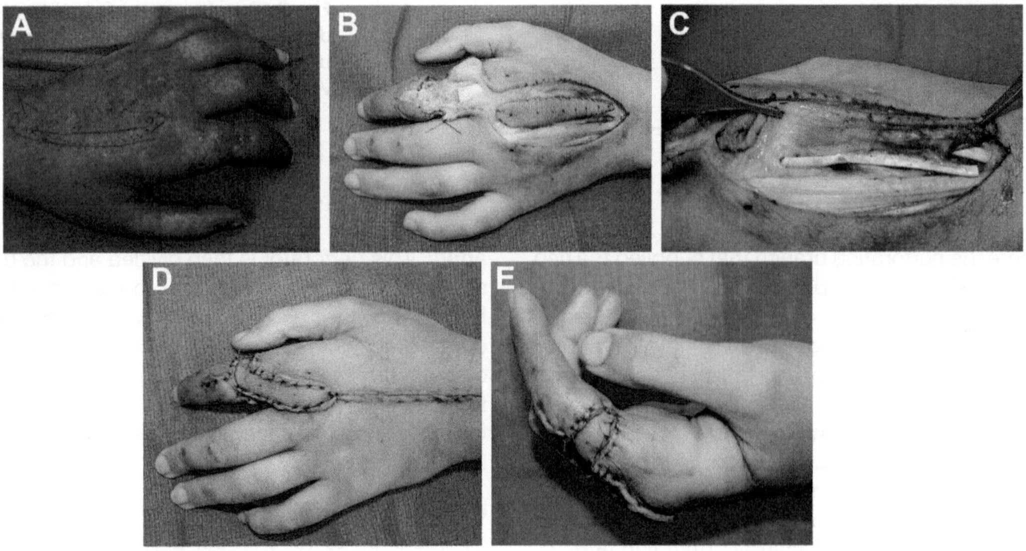

Fig. 10. (*A–E*) A case using vascularized tendon.

move more distally like the modification described by Karacalar and Özcan.

Donor Sites

For donor sites often a split thickness sheet graft can be used rather than a full thickness graft. The dorsal hand tolerates the graft contracture well and this minimizes the donor site morbidity.

DISCLOSURE

The authors have nothing to disclose.

SUPPLEMENTARY DATA

Supplementary data related to this article can be found online at https://doi.org/10.1016/j.hcl.2019.09.001.

REFERENCES

1. Littler JW. The neurovascular pedicle method of digital transposition for reconstruction of the thumb. Plast Reconstr Surg (1946) 1953;12(5):303–19. Available at: http://www.ncbi.nlm.nih.gov/pubmed/13111910.
2. Hilgenfeld O. Operativer Daumenersatz Und Beseitigung von Greifstörungen Bei Fingerverlusten. Stuttgart: Enke; 1950.
3. Holevich J. A new method of restoring sensibility to the thumb. J Bone Joint Surg Br 1963;45:496–502. Available at: http://www.ncbi.nlm.nih.gov/pubmed/14058323.
4. Holevitch Y. Use of skin islet flap from the dorsal aspect of index finger for restoration of the sensitivity in the thumb. Acta Chir Plast 1964;6:1–8. Available at: http://www.ncbi.nlm.nih.gov/pubmed/14134960.
5. Lie KK, Posch JL. Island flap innervated by radial nerve for restoration of sensation in an index stump. Case report. Plast Reconstr Surg 1971;47(4):386–8. Available at: http://www.ncbi.nlm.nih.gov/pubmed/4927278.
6. Foucher G, Braun JB. A new island flap transfer from the dorsum of the index to the thumb. Plast Reconstr Surg 1979;63(3):344–9. Available at: http://www.ncbi.nlm.nih.gov/pubmed/368837.
7. Adachi B, Hasebe K. Das Arteriensystem Der Japaner. Kyoto: Kaiserlich-Japanischen Universitat zu Kyoto; 1928. p. 20–71.
8. Lister G. The theory of the transposition flap and its practical application in the hand. Clin Plast Surg 1981;8(1):115–27. Available at: http://www.ncbi.nlm.nih.gov/pubmed/7273610.
9. Earley MJ. The arterial supply of the thumb, first web and index finger and its surgical application. J Hand Surg Br 1986;11(2):163–74. Available at: http://www.ncbi.nlm.nih.gov/pubmed/3734551.
10. Earley MJ, Milner RH. Dorsal metacarpal flaps. Br J Plast Surg 1987;40(4):333–41. Available at: http://www.ncbi.nlm.nih.gov/pubmed/3620777.
11. Quaba A, Davison P. The distally-based dorsal hand flap. Br J Plast Surg 1990;43(1):28–39.
12. Maruyama Y. The reverse dorsal metacarpal flap. Br J Plast Surg 1990;43(1):24–7.
13. Yang D, Morris SF. Vascular basis of dorsal digital and metacarpal skin flaps. J Hand Surg Am 2001;26(1):142–6.
14. Santa-Comba A, Amarante J, Silva Á, et al. Reverse dorsal metacarpal osteocutaneous flap. Br J Plast Surg 1997;50(7):555–8.

15. Sherif MM. First dorsal metacarpal artery flap in hand reconstruction. I. Anatomical study. J Hand Surg Am 1994;19(1):26–31.
16. Karacalar A, Ozcan M. A new approach to the reverse dorsal metacarpal artery flap. J Hand Surg Am 1997;22(2):307–10.
17. Gebhard B, Meissl G. An extended first dorsal metacarpal artery neurovascular island flap. J Hand Surg Br 1995;20B(4):529–31.
18. El-Khatib HA. Clinical experiences with the extended first dorsal metacarpal artery island flap for thumb reconstruction. J Hand Surg Am 1998;23(4):647–52.
19. Yao JM, Song JL, Xu JH. The second web bilobed island flap for thumb reconstruction. Br J Plast Surg 1996;49(2):103–6.
20. Small JO, Brennen MD. The first dorsal metacarpal artery neurovascular island flap. J Hand Surg Br 1988;13(2):136–45. Available at: http://www.ncbi.nlm.nih.gov/pubmed/3385287.
21. Foucher G, Braun FM, Merle M, et al. La technique du "de branchment-rebranchment" due lambear enilot pedicule. Ann Chir 1981;35(4): 301–3.
22. Earley MJ. The second dorsal metacarpal artery neurovascular island flap. J Hand Surg Br 1989; 14(4):434–40. Available at: http://www.ncbi.nlm.nih.gov/pubmed/2482855.
23. Karacalar A, Akin S, Özcan M. The second dorsal metacarpal artery flap with double pivot points. Br J Plast Surg 1996;49(2):97–102.

Free Flaps for Soft Tissue Reconstruction of Digits

Yohan Lee, MD[a], Sang-Hyun Woo, MD, PhD[b], Young-Woo Kim, MD, PhD[b], Young Ho Lee, MD, PhD[c,*], Goo Hyun Baek, MD, PhD[c,*]

KEYWORDS

• Free flap • Finger • Digits • Reconstruction • Microsurgery

KEY POINTS

- Soft tissue reconstruction in the digits is challenging for hand surgeons because both functional and aesthetic aspects must be considered.
- A satisfactory outcome can be achieved by performing thorough debridement, reliable flap coverage, and beginning joint motion at an early stage.
- Free flap is recommended when the defect is too large for coverage with a local flap, when there are defects on multiple digits, or when the defect is associated with loss of other structures that need reconstruction.
- Proper flap selection is essential depending on the location and function of the digits. The key to flap selection is to maintain similarity to the missing tissue.
- Partial toe pulp flap is best suited for fingertip reconstruction because it provides durable and glabrous skin with good sensibility and aesthetic appearance.

The primary cause of soft tissue defects of the digits is work-related trauma. Hands and digits are the most frequently treated body parts in the emergency room, owing to injury while working.[1] In the United States, at least 1 million workers visit hospitals owing to injury to the digits and hands each year.[2] Four to 11 of every 100 workers have received treatment of their hands and digit injuries.[3] There are a variety of available treatment options for digital defects, such as healing by secondary intention, primary closure, skin grafts, local advancement flaps, local pedicled flaps, and free flaps.[4] Hand surgeons must select a treatment option considering the condition of the wound, concomitant injuries, underlying disease, and patient circumstances (eg, socioeconomic status and cultural background). During treatment of digital injuries, functional limitations and poor outcomes arise as a result of prolonged immobilization and multiple operations. Therefore, even if the surgical method is complex, a better outcome is likely to be achieved by performing aggressive treatment from the beginning.[5,6]

Tendons and bones are closely related to the skin especially on the dorsum of the digits and are easily exposed or damaged by trauma. Treatment with skin grafts or local flaps has limitations in certain clinical situations, and a free flap can be considered in the following situations[7]:

1. When the defect is too large to cover with a local flap, or when there are multiple defects.
2. When options for local flaps are within the zone of trauma and the vascular integrity cannot be guaranteed.

Disclosure: The authors have nothing to disclose.

[a] Department of Orthopaedic Surgery, Seoul National University Boramae Hospital, 20, Boramae-ro 5-gil, Dongjak-gu, Seoul 07061, Republic of Korea; [b] W Institute for Hand and Reconstructive Microsurgery, W Hospital, 1632 Dalgubeol-daero, Dalseo-Gu, Daegu 42642, Republic of Korea; [c] Department of Orthopaedic Surgery, Seoul National University Hospital, 101, Daehak-ro, Jongno-gu, Seoul 03080, Republic of Korea

* Corresponding authors.

E-mail addresses: orthoyhl@snu.ac.kr (Y.H.L.); ghbaek@snu.ac.kr (G.H.B.)

Hand Clin 36 (2020) 85–96

https://doi.org/10.1016/j.hcl.2019.08.008

3. When a local flap cannot be attempted because of vascular abnormality.
4. When simultaneous reconstruction of complex structures (eg, bone, tendon, and/or nerve) is required.

GENERAL PRINCIPLES

Preoperative Considerations

Detailed history-taking and sufficient discussion with patients help to generate a comprehensive treatment plan. Significant past medical history should be noted and addressed, where possible, for factors such as peripheral vascular disease, diabetes, and smoking, which may affect the survival of the flap. In addition, patient occupation and age are important factors that can affect postoperative satisfaction and the survival of the flap. The choice of a donor site in a free flap is essential. If the reason for selection of the donor site is not fully explained to patients, there may be greater dissatisfaction with donor site morbidity. Hand surgeons should discuss the treatment goals, available treatment options, and expected complications with their patients. All flaps have a possibility of failure. Before the first operation and during treatment, surgeons should discuss with their patients regarding second-line treatments, which can be performed if current treatment fails or unintended consequences occur. This discussion should be documented, and patient consent should be obtained.

Imaging studies are recommended because the vascular system can exhibit considerable variation. Preoperative confirmation of the integrity of target vessels of donor and recipient sites should be performed by computed tomography (CT) angiography. Doppler sonography should be used to check the perforator flap, compare it with the angiography image, and mark the exact location on the skin. In the operating room, the surgeon should prepare Doppler sonography for localization of the perforator during surgery.

Assessment of associated injury is essential. Active and passive motion of a joint should be tested routinely to determine whether tendon injury has occurred. Radiography is used as a first-line assessment to detect fractures. If necessary, CT can be used for confirmation. If a deep infection is suspected, MRI can be useful.

Debridement

Sufficient debridement is necessary to increase the chances of survival of the flap and reduce the occurrence of complications.[8–11] Debridement reduces the bacterial load and distinguishes structures that can be preserved so that an appropriate reconstruction plan can be developed.[12] Debridement can be performed in the emergency room, but is ideally done under tourniquet control in the operating room under aseptic conditions. After sufficient irrigation with normal saline, all nonviable tissues are removed by using a scalpel or scissors. After debridement, wound characteristics should be noted and recorded, including the depth, width, location, boundary, and status of the wound bed, as well as whether there is neurovascular, bone or tendon injury.

Neurovascular structures should be dissected after debridement. There is some controversy with regards to choosing the site of anastomosis with some investigators reporting good outcomes in the zone of trauma as well as distal to the zone of trauma.[13–16] The authors prefer to perform the arterial repair proximal to the zone of trauma. If the anastomosis site is too proximal and cannot reach the perforator, an interposition vein graft can be considered. However, another possible option is anastomosis distal to the zone of trauma, if patency is determined in the operating room. This selection depends on the surgeon's preference.

In the past, it was recommended to perform definite reconstruction within 24 to 72 hours after soft tissue injury occurred. Recently, however, studies have shown that there is no difference in outcomes, even if subacute reconstruction is performed after 72 hours. If the distinction between viable and nonviable tissue is clear, or if neurovascular structure is exposed, reconstruction should be conducted immediately after debridement. If the boundary of the viable tissue is ambiguous or the tissue shows signs of infection, serial debridement (over several days) should be performed to distinguish the edges of the viable tissue. A sterile and wet environment should be maintained between phases of serial debridement by using occlusive dressing or negative pressure dressing. However, care should be taken when using negative pressure dressing, because it can occasionally cause severe pain. The authors prefer to perform reconstruction of the digit within 1 week after injury.

Flap Selection

Digital skin has a unique structure. The dorsum is thin and elastic, facilitating joint motion, whereas the palmar tissue is thick and sturdy to perform manual tasks. The fingertip provides sensibility and ensures that the digit functions correctly.[4] The key principles of soft tissue reconstruction in the digit are to restore tissue that is similar to the missing tissue, maintain mobility, and provide as much sensory recovery as possible.[6] The free flaps that are suitable for this role are listed in **Table 1**.

Postoperative Care and Rehabilitation

The patients are given a once-daily dose of enoxaparin (Clexane; Sanofi-Aventis, Paris, France) 40 mg subcutaneously and alprostadil (Eglandin; Mitsubishi Tanabe, Osaka, Japan) 10 μg intravenously for 7 days after surgery. Flap viability is evaluated by monitoring capillary refill, color, surface temperature, and swelling. The flap monitoring is checked twice per day until 7 days after surgery. If the survival of the flap is ambiguous, Doppler sonography or flap bleeding can be used for verification. If the flap is stable, joint motion can be started gradually from the first week after the surgery.

SPECIFIC FLAPS

Partial Toe Pulp Flap

A pulp defect of the fingertip is difficult to reconstruct because of its functional and structural specificity. The pulp skin is anchored by fibrous septa extending from the periosteum to the dermis that allows it to withstand mechanical stress. The septae enclose the subcutaneous fat, thus providing a stable surface for grip and pinch. In addition, the pulp has a high concentration of Meissner and Pacinian neurosensory receptors, providing keen sensibility.[4,30] Although a neurorrhaphy has been described for a variety of flaps used in fingertip reconstruction, the sensory recovery is inevitably poor, simply because these flaps have fewer neurosensory receptors than pulp. The unique anatomy of the pulp is the rationale for using a "like-for-like" reconstructive approach for fingertip flap reconstruction[31]

In 1979, Buncke and Rose[17] introduced reconstruction of the fingertip using partial toe pulp. When first introduced, the success rate was approximately 60%, which was not superior to that of other reconstructive options. This pattern continued until the early 1990s.[32] However, with the development of better microsurgical techniques, success rates have continued to increase and have reached an average of 98%.[18,33–35]

Toe pulp flaps are advantageous in that they can provide a "like-for-like" reconstruction with a durable and glabrous flap, with texture similar to that of the lost tissue. In addition, toe pulp flaps exhibit excellent sensory recovery and high aesthetic satisfaction for both donor and recipient sites. Therefore, the partial toe pulp flap is the authors' preferred tissue for reconstruction of the fingertip (**Fig. 1**).[18]

Indication

The authors use the toe pulp flap for finger and thumb tip reconstruction. A partial great toe pulp flap can measure up to 4.5 cm in length and 2.5 cm in width, whereas a second toe pulp flap can measure up to 3 cm in length and 2.5 cm in width.[18,31,36] The size of the flap relative to the toe is more important than the total flap size, because toe size varies among individuals. For linear closure of the donor site, the width of the flap must be limited to less than half the width of the donor toe pulp.[37]

Surgical Anatomy

The donor used in the partial toe pulp transfer is the lateral (fibular) surface of the great toe and the medial (tibial) surface of the second toe. The authors base their flaps on a short pedicle that includes the plantar digital arteries and plantar digital nerve. There is controversy over the vein that should be used in the flap.[38] Initially, the superficial dorsal vein was used; however, its failure rate was high because of difficulty in harvesting it in continuity with the flap.[39] Lee and colleagues[18] in their large series of 929 second toe pulp transfers used a plantar subcutaneous vein in a short pedicle transfer. Sun and colleagues[40] suggested the use of the accompanying vein as a draining vein, instead of a superficial dorsal vein. They also suggested harvesting the toe web space communicating branch between the accompanying veins and the dorsal metatarsal veins. Communicating branch of toe web veins made it possible to anastomose the larger-caliber dorsal metatarsal vein instead of the thin accompanying vein.

Operating Technique

Surgery is performed with the patient supine under general anesthesia and with tourniquet control. The size of the fingertip defect is measured after adequate debridement. An additional volar zig-zag incision is made proximal to the defect in order to dissect the neurovascular bundle. Caution is needed to avoid damaging the subcutaneous veins while making the incision. A flap is designed in the toe pulp based on the size and shape of the defect. An additional zig-zag incision is made to detect the vessels proximal to the flap. When harvesting the toe pulp, a 2-mm section of skin near the eponychial fold must be left to prevent nail-related problems.[18] On the proximal side of the flap, 1 or more subcutaneous veins are identified by subdermal dissection. There are often 1 or 2 subcutaneous veins in the flap,

Table 1
Considerations for free-flap reconstruction in the digits

Free Flap	Blood Supply	Innervation	Indications	Advantages	Disadvantages
Toe pulp flap[17,18]	Plantar digital artery	Plantar proper digital nerve	Fingertip	Cosmetic satisfaction; durable and glabrous skin, improved sensory recovery	Donor site morbidity
Thenar flap[19,20]	Superficial palmar branch of radial artery	Lateral antebrachial cutaneous nerve, superficial sensory branch of the radial nerve	Palmar aspect	Durable	Variable nerve distribution
RASP flap[20,21]	Superficial palmar branch of radial artery	Palmar cutaneous branch of the median nerve	Palmar aspect	Constant anatomy (nerve), durable, innervated	Small size
Anterolateral thigh flap[22,23]	Descending branch of the medial femoral circumflex artery	None	Anywhere	For large defects or multiple defects; easy to design	Thick, less aesthetic satisfaction, less sensitivity
First web space flap[24]	First dorsal metatarsal artery, plantar digital artery	Deep peroneal nerve, medial plantar nerve	Anywhere	Glabrous skin, better sensory recovery	Anatomic variation, difficulty of dissection
Wrap-around free flap[25]	Medial and lateral plantar digital artery	Medial and lateral plantar digital nerve	Ring avulsion injury	Soft tissue reconstruction with nail bed	Donor site morbidity
Medial plantar flap[26]	Medial or lateral plantar artery	Medial plantar nerve	Fingertip, palmar aspect	Durable, glabrous skin	Thick, donor site morbidity
Dorsalis pedis flap[27,28]	Dorsalis pedis artery, first dorsal metatarsal artery	Superficial peroneal nerve	Anywhere	Donor site morbidity	Less sensitivity
Venous flap[29]	Variable	Variable	Dorsal and lateral of proximal phalanx, palmar aspect	Used for large defects or multiple defects	Possibility of partial necrosis

Data from Refs.[17–29]

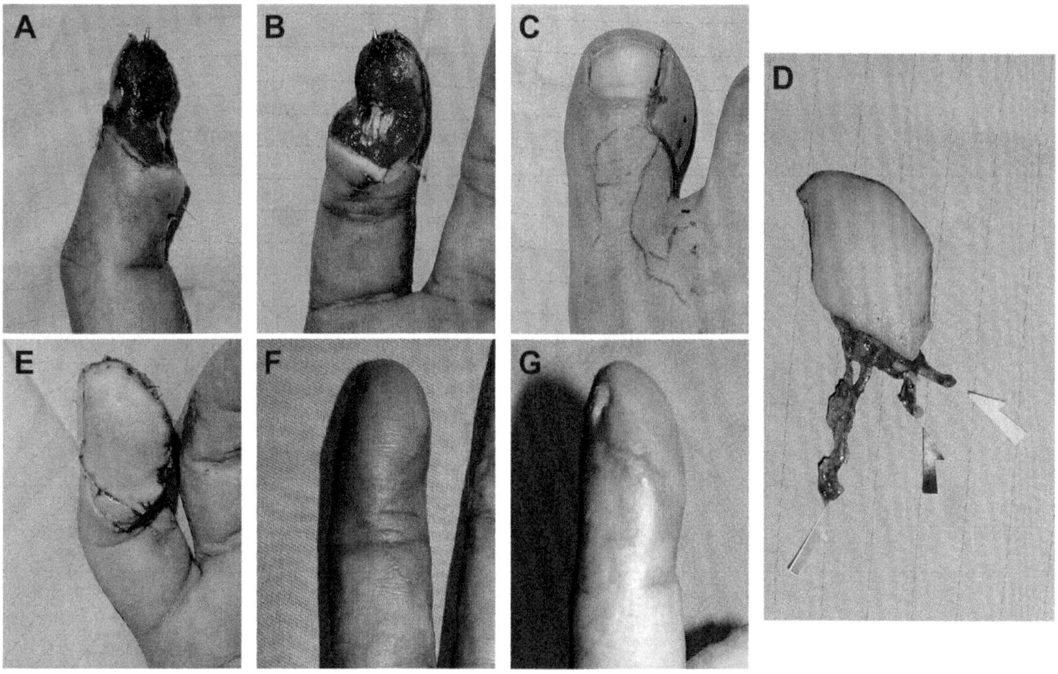

Fig. 1. (*A*, *B*) Preoperative views of pulp defect of the left index finger. (*C*) Design of the pulp flap on the lateral aspect of the great toe. (*D*) Dissected pulp flap with digital artery (*red arrow*), subcutaneous vein (*blue arrow*), and digital nerve (*yellow arrow*). (*E*) Immediate postoperative view. (*F*, *G*) Eight months postoperatively.

but these vary in size from 0.8 mm to 2 mm. Elevation of the flap is started after the vein is located. Dissection of the flap is performed through the pretendinous layer. During dissection in a distal to proximal direction, the vertical fibers distributed in the pulp are released. As flap elevation proceeds, the surgeon can locate the plantar digital artery and accompanying vein below the flap. The proper plantar digital nerve is also dissected for neurorrhaphy. When the dissection continues proximally, the communicating branch to another plantar digital artery can be found near the proximal interphalangeal joint. The communicating branch is ligated while avoiding damage to the main vessel. When the harvested pedicle is sufficiently long for transfer to the defect, the tourniquet is released, and flap circulation is checked. If the circulation is intact, the pedicle is cut, and the flap is transferred to the recipient site. Anastomosis of neurovascular structures between donor and recipient is performed. The digital artery of the toe pulp is typically matched in size with the digital artery at the level of the middle phalanx level of the finger.[18] After neurorrhaphy and vessel anastomosis, the digital skin is sutured without tension. The direct closure of the donor toe often results in a pale appearance of the toe. Circulation typically returns within 1 hour. If the pale appearance persists after 1 hour, a skin graft can be used to cover a portion of the wound after selected suture removal.

Outcomes

Partial toe pulp flap is a technically challenging procedure. If the surgeon is proficient in microsurgical techniques, a good outcome can be achieved. The success rate of partial toe pulp flap is recently reported to be 99.7% to 100%. Two-point discrimination is achieved from 4 to 15 (**Table 2**).[17,18,33,40]

Radial Artery Superficial Palmar Branch Flap

The thenar area is glabrous and has similar characteristics to the palmar side of the fingers, making it suitable for use in small flaps. The first attempt to use a thenar flap was in the 1990s by Tsai and colleagues[19] and Kamei and colleagues,[20] who used a flap based on the superficial branch of the radial artery for finger reconstruction. The initial description of this flap was a skin flap without a nerve included. Subsequently, a sensate thenar flap was attempted using either a branch of the lateral antebrachial cutaneous nerve or the superficial radial nerve. However, these branches were not consistent, and the sensate thenar flap did not become popular.[41,42] Sakai[21] developed a flap

Table 2
Outcomes of partial toe pulp flap

Authors, Year	Number of Subjects	Defect Size (cm)	Vein Source in the Flap	Survival Rate (%)	Static Two-Point Discrimination (mm) (Mean)	Complications
Buncke & Rose,[17] 1979	6	Not mentioned	Superficial dorsal digital vein	66.7 (4/6)	3–7 (4.5)	2 Complete failures
Lee et al,[18] 2008	929	2.7 × 1.7–3.3 × 2.3	Plantar subcutaneous vein	99.7 (926/929)	4–15 (8)	72 Arterial spasm of recipient site 39 Hematomas of donor site 20 Wounds dehiscence of donor site
Kimura,[33] 2009	27	1 × 2–3 × 6	Plantar subcutaneous vein	100 (27/27)	4–15 (9)	2 Arterial insufficiency of donor site
Sun et al,[40] 2010	14	2.0 × 1.5–4.0 × 1.5	Communicating branch of the toe web vein	100 (14/14)	Not mentioned	Not mentioned

Data from Refs.[17,18,33,40]

that used the palmar cutaneous branch of the median nerve and superficial palmar branch of the radial artery in 2003. This flap is known as the radial artery superficial palmar branch (RASP) flap. The main advantage of this flap is the consistent nerve and arterial anatomy (**Fig. 2**).[42]

Indication

Although the RASP flap can be applied to any part of the finger, it is mainly recommended for use in fingertip and palmar defects, because of the tissue similarity.[42] For fingertip defects, an RASP flap can be considered if the defects are too large for

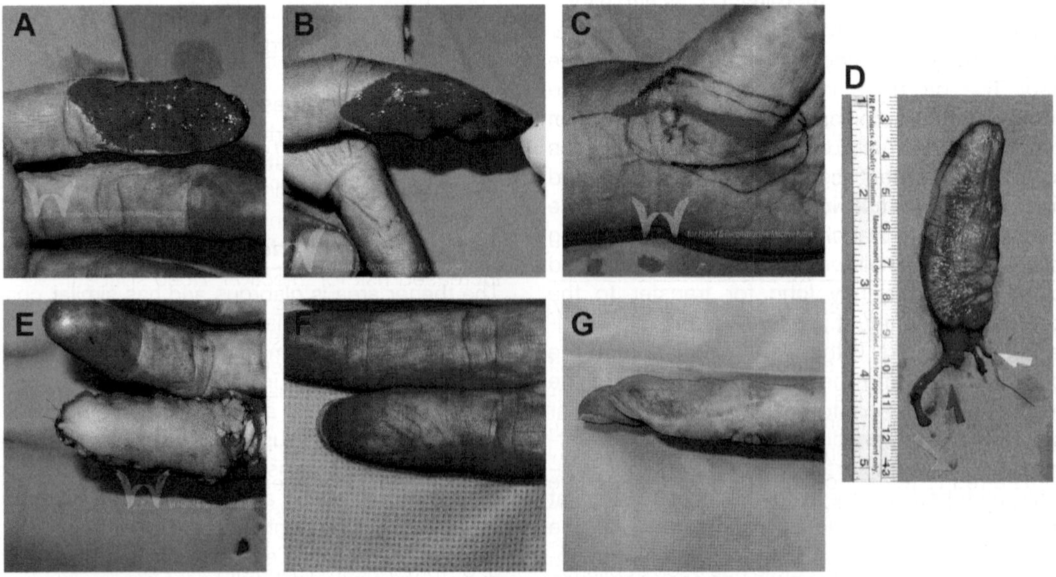

Fig. 2. (*A, B*) Preoperative view of a volar soft tissue defect of the left index finger: distal and middle phalanx. (*C*) Design of the RASP flap on the palm side of the left hand. (*D*) Dissected RASP flap with radial artery superficial branch (*red arrow*), accompanying vein of radial artery (*blue arrow*), and palmar cutaneous branch of the median nerve (*yellow arrow*). (*E*) Immediate postoperative view. (*F, G*) Five years postoperatively.

coverage by a partial toe pulp flap, or if the patient is not agreeable to toe flaps. An RASP flap of dimensions of up to 3 cm in width and 8 cm in length has been described.[42,43]

Surgical Anatomy

In a study of 30 cadavers, Yang and colleagues[42] performed a detailed examination of the location of the palmar cutaneous branch of the median nerve and superficial palmar branch of the radial artery. Based on their findings, they suggested a proper flap design and placement for the RASP flap. The palmar cutaneous branch of the median nerve was present in all cadavers in the study, arising from the median nerve in the distal one-third of the forearm, ulnar side to the flexor carpi radialis. This branch reaches the skin of the interthenar area at the level of the distal wrist crease after piercing the antebrachial fascia. This area is within approximately 3 cm of the radial styloid and scaphoid tuberosity. Occasionally, branches from the lateral antebrachial cutaneous nerve or superficial radial nerve can be included in the flap; however, their presence is not consistent.

Yang and colleagues[42] reported that the superficial palmar branch of the radial artery originated at a mean of 11.56 $\pm$ 4.32 mm from the radial styloid process. Its average diameter was 1.49 $\pm$ 0.46 mm at its origin and matches the digital artery. The superficial palmar branch of the radial artery provides vascular supply to the skin overlying the scaphoid tuberosity. This branch then enters the thenar muscles. Independent skin branches, separated from thenar muscle branches, were present in only 13.3% of the cadavers analyzed in their study.[42] This flap is best designed longitudinally and centered over the scaphoid tuberosity.

Operative Technique

Surgery is performed with the patient in the supine position under general anesthesia and with tourniquet control. After debridement, the size of the defect is measured. A longitudinally elliptical flap is designed in the interthenar area overlying the scaphoid tuberosity. An additional incision is made in the proximal part of the flap to allow dissection of vascular structures. In the proximal part, the skin flaps are raised in a subdermal plane to avoid injury to the subcutaneous veins. One or more superficial veins are typically present in the proximal portion of the flap. The superficial branch of the radial artery can be located in a plane deeper to the veins. The radial side of the flap is dissected, and the branch of the thenar muscle is located and ligated. The distal and ulnar part of the flap is then dissected. The palmar cutaneous branch of the median nerve can be found in the proximal ulnar side of the flap. Once an adequate length of pedicle is obtained, the tourniquet is released, and flap perfusion is assessed. The pedicle is then divided; the flap is transferred to the recipient site, and microvascular repair is performed to the digital artery, vein, and nerve. The donor vein is typically anastomosed to a palmar digital vein. If there are no suitable veins on the palmar side, a dorsal digital vein can be used as the recipient vein. If there are signs of congestion after anastomosis, the accompanying vein can also be repaired. The flap is inset without tension once the microsurgical procedures are complete.

Outcomes

The success rate of RASP flap is reported to be 91% to 100%. A 2-point discrimination of 7 to 13 mm with neurorrhaphy, and from 10 to 16 mm without neurorrhaphy, has been reported (**Table 3**).[43–47]

Arterialized Venous Flap

The arterialized venous flap comprises both afferent and efferent vessels, along with veins. This concept was first introduced in 1981 by Nakayama and colleagues.[29] The most important advantage of an arterialized venous flap is that it allows thin and pliable flaps to be obtained without sacrificing a critical artery. Theoretically, there is no limit to the choice of the flap donor site because the venous network can be located in any part of the skin of the body.[48] The disadvantage of the venous flap is that the outcome is unpredictable because the circulation is not physiologic. The overall survival of the flap is similar to that of other free flaps.[48,49] However, close monitoring is necessary because there is a risk of venous congestion, epidermolysis, and marginal necrosis.[48,50]

Flap survival is based on blood supply and tissue perfusion via the venous network, because the blood does not flow through a physiologic artery-arteriole-capillary-venule-vein system. Therefore, the flap should be designed over skin with a well-developed venous network (**Fig. 3**). Free venous flaps can be divided into 3 categories depending on the recipient vessel type.[50] In the first type, there is total venous perfusion with both afferent and efferent vein connected to the recipient and donor vein, respectively (V-V-V). In the second type, there is total arterial perfusion with the afferent and efferent vein connected to the recipient and

Table 3
Outcomes of radial artery superficial palmar branch flap

Authors, Year	Number of Subjects	Flap Size (cm)	Survival Rate (%)	Static Two-Point Discrimination (mm) (Mean)	Complications
Chi et al,[43] 2018	79	Not mentioned	100 (79/79)	7–13	1 Partial necrosis
Lee et al,[44] 2017	125	2 × 1–3.5 × 7	91.2 (114/125)	With neurorrhaphy: 10–13 (12) Without neurorrhaphy: 10–16 (13)	4 Hypertrophic scars on donor site 1 Pillar pain on donor site
Zhang et al,[45] 2015	14	2.8 × 2.0–4.5 × 2.5	100 (14/14)	26–14 (9.7)	2 Wound infections 1 Venous congestion
Iwuagwu et al,[46] 2015	13	2 × 5–2 × 10	100 (13/13)	6–8 (6.7)	6 Flap revisions
Lee et al,[47] 2009	11	2.4 × 1.2–5.0 × 2.5	100 (11/11)	9–11 (8.8)	1 Partial necrosis 1 Scar band contracture 1 Joint stiffness

Data from Refs.[43–47]

donor artery, respectively (A-V-A). Total venous perfusion and total arterial perfusion venous flaps are both connected to the same recipient vessel structure, but the direction of afferent and efferent blood flow must be maintained. In such cases, the flap acts as a conduit for connection between veins or arteries. The third type of free venous flap is the arterialized venous flap. Here, an artery is connected to the afferent vein, and a vein is connected to the efferent vein (A-V-V).

Indication

The most important consideration in the survival of the venous flaps is perfusion. Woo and colleagues[48] recommended that a venous flap be used for small defects and for defects that are located proximally. The perfusion of the skin decreases as one moves away from the vein, so survival of smaller flaps is better compared with larger flaps. Also, the blood flow in the digit is weaker as one moves distally. The V-V-V flap is typically used

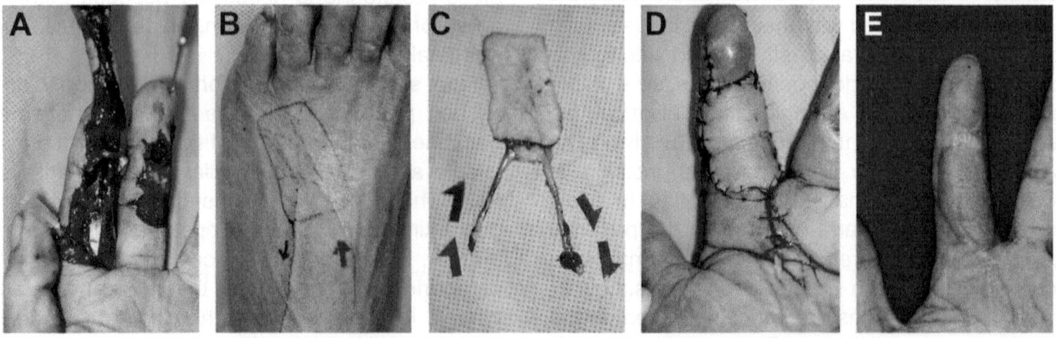

Fig. 3. (*A*) Volar aspect of the left index finger, which was avulsed distally by a galvanized steel sheet. This caused soft tissue loss with intact flexor tendon. (*B*) Venous flap that was designed on the dorsal aspect of the foot, approximately 2 cm × 4.5 cm. (*C*) The venous flap was harvested with 2 veins. One afferent vein was anastomosed to the ulnar digital artery of the index (*red arrow*), and 1 efferent vein was sutured to the dorsal subcutaneous vein (*blue arrows*). (*D*, *E*) Views immediately after surgery and 6 months postoperatively.

for defects overlying the proximal phalanx. An A-V-A flap can be used anywhere on the digit provided a distal artery is available. However, it is not recommended for pulp defects because of durability and sensory limitations. The condition of the recipient bed is also important in the survival of free venous flaps. Support of the surrounding tissue is necessary to increase the rate of survival. If the bone is exposed and the flap is placed directly on the bone, or there is infection, the flap survival rate will be lowered.

Surgical Anatomy

Careful consideration of the condition of the venous network and selection of the donor site is essential because venous congestion is the major cause of failure. Anatomic considerations comprise the direction of the flow and the length, number, and size of the afferent and efferent veins.

Woo and colleagues[48] described a classification approach according to the shape of the venous network and the direction of the flow and suggested venous flap designs for different types of soft tissue defects. They recommended that the best perfusion was achieved by repairing both the artery and the vein in the direction of the flow. However, if this could not be done, the artery could be anastomosed to a vein against the direction of flow, but the vein must be anastomosed in the direction of flow. In such a situation, the length of the afferent vein should be minimized to decrease blood flow interference by the valves. If the venous network has several veins, there should be at least 1 efferent vein with the valve in the forward direction. The size of the efferent vein should be larger than that of the afferent vein. The number of veins should also be considered. Generally, there should be more efferent veins than afferent veins. Greater numbers of veins, relative to circulation, should be considered as the flap size increases. The authors recommended that a small-sized flap (<10 cm^2) should have at least 1 afferent vein and 1 efferent vein; a medium-sized flap (10–25 cm^2) should have at least 1 afferent vein and 2 efferent veins, and a large-sized flap (>25 cm^2) should have at least 2 afferent veins and 2 or more efferent veins.[48] Theoretically, there is no limit regarding the choice of the donor site. The authors of this article prefer to harvest from the volar aspect of the forearm in the same limb as the defect, or from the dorsum of the foot. In either location, the venous network is well developed and easy to detect, and the skin is thin.

Operative Technique

Nonviable tissue is completely debrided. The flap is designed with consideration of the size and shape of the defect. In situations where innervated venous flaps are used, a flap with a dorsal cutaneous nerve of the foot can be used for reconstruction of palmar defects of the digit.[48] When performing a tendon reconstruction together with the flap surgery, a segment of the palmaris longus may be harvested in combination with the arterialized venous flap in the forearm.[51] If there are multiple adjacent digital defects, a large arterialized venous flap can be used after the digits are syndactylized surgically. The syndactyly is divided 5 to 6 weeks later, once the flap is stable.[48]

A pneumatic tourniquet at a pressure of 75 to 100 mm Hg is applied. This pneumatic tourniquet interrupts the venous return, making the venous network engorged. The venous network under the skin is then marked with a pen. The flap is designed such that the venous network is located in the center of the flap. The location and number of afferent and efferent veins are selected. The length of the afferent vein is as short as possible, and the length of the efferent vein is determined with respect to the location of the recipient vessel. The flap typically consists of only skin, including subcutaneous tissue, and veins without fascia. However, the configuration of the flap is not always constant. Depending on the defect site, the bone or tendons can be included in the flap.[48,51] When flap dissection is complete, the flap is transferred to the defect, and anastomosis is performed. The lowest possible number of skin sutures is used, without tension. Venous flaps show severe edema and discoloration, compared with other free flaps in early postoperative stages. This phenomenon may be caused by changes in direction of blood flow by the valves.[48] Edema and discoloration improve gradually over the next few weeks.

Outcomes

The venous flap survival rate is similar or slightly lower than that of other free flaps. The success rate of arterialized venous flap is reported to be 75% to 98.1% (**Table 4**).[48,49,52–54] There are several factors involved in the survival of venous flaps. Chen and colleagues[50] reported that venous flaps with total venous perfusion have lower rates of survival than other types of flaps. Woo and colleagues[46] reported that a higher number of draining vessels was associated with a higher rate of survival and lower rate of partial necrosis. The size of the flap is also an important factor. Generally, large venous flaps should not be used in fingers or hand, although the size of such flaps has not shown a significant correlation with survival in the hand. Poor vascularity of the recipient site can also reduce the success rate.

Table 4
Outcomes of arterialized venous flap

Authors, Year	Number of Subjects	Donor Site	Survival Rate (%)	Flap Size	Composition of Vessels (Afferent-Flap-Efferent)	Number of Anastomosis (Afferent-Efferent)	Complications
Park et al,[52] 2015	12	Distal volar forearm	75 (9/12)	1 × 1.5–5 × 7 cm	A-V-V	7 (1–1) 3 (1–2) 1 (2–2) 1 (1–3)	3 Partial necrosis
Kayalar et al,[53] 2014	41	39 Forearm, 1 dorsum of hand, 1 saphenous vein	90.2 (37/41)	2 × 1.5–3 × 10 cm	36 A-V-V 5 A-V-A	14 (1-1) 18 (1-2) 9 (2-2)	4 Total necrosis
Kong et al,[54] 2008	44	Distal volar forearm	88.6 (39/44)	1 × 1–5.5 × 4.5 cm	A-V-V	40 (1-1) 3 (1-2) 1 (2-1)	5 Total necrosis
Woo et al,[48] 2007	154	93 Volar forearm 37 Thenar area/volar aspect of the wrist 16 Dorsum of the foot 8 Medial aspect of the calf	98.1 (151/154)	48 Small (<10 cm^2) 64 Medium (10–25 cm^2) 42 Large (>25 cm^2)	A-V-V A-V-V A-V-V	$(1.04 \pm 0.20–1.13 \pm 0.33)$[a] $(1.19 \pm 0.39–1.41 \pm 0.50)$[a] $(1.79 \pm 0.42–2.29 \pm 0.60)$[a]	2 Partial necrosis 1 Flap failure 2 Partial necrosis 1 Flap failure 4 Partial necrosis

Abbreviations: A, artery; V, vein.
[a] Only mean numbers of vessels are provided.
Data from Refs.[48,52–54]

SUMMARY

Soft tissue construction in the finger is challenging for hand surgeons because both functional and aesthetic aspects must be considered. A satisfactory outcome can be achieved by initiating joint motion at an early stage following adequate debridement and reliable flap coverage. A free flap is recommended when the defect is too large for coverage with a local flap, when there are defects on multiple fingers, or when the defect is present with other damaged structures. Proper flap selection is essential depending on the location and function of the fingers. The key to flap selection is to maintain similarity to the missing tissue. Partial toe pulp flaps are considered the primary choice of treatment of fingertip reconstruction because it has a durable and glabrous texture with a keen sensibility and aesthetic benefit. The advantage of RASP flaps is constant nerve and vascular anatomy that can be applied as a sensate flap on a moderate-sized defect of the palmar side of a finger. An arterialized venous flap offers the benefit of easily harvested thin and pliable flaps without sacrificing a critical artery.

REFERENCES

1. Centers for Disease Control and Prevention. Surveillance for nonfatal occupational injuries treated in hospital emergency departments–United States, 1996. MMWR Morb Mortal Wkly Rep 1998;47(15): 302–6.
2. Sorock GS, Lombardi DA, Hauser RB, et al. Acute traumatic occupational hand injuries: type, location, and severity. J Occup Environ Med 2002;44(4): 345–51.
3. Sorock GS, Lombardi DA, Courtney TK, et al. Epidemiology of occupational acute traumatic hand injuries: a literature review. Saf Sci 2001;38(3):241–56.
4. Yannascoli SM, Thibaudeau S, Levin LS. Management of soft tissue defects of the hand. J Hand Surg Am 2015;40(6):1237–44 [quiz: 1245].
5. Gottlieb LJ, Krieger LM. From the reconstructive ladder to the reconstructive elevator. Plast Reconstr Surg 1994;93(7):1503–4.
6. Miller EA, Friedrich J. Soft tissue coverage of the hand and upper extremity: the reconstructive elevator. J Hand Surg Am 2016;41(7):782–92.
7. Saint-Cyr M, Gupta A. Indications and selection of free flaps for soft tissue coverage of the upper extremity. Hand Clin 2007;23(1):37–48.
8. Lister G, Scheker L. Emergency free flaps to the upper extremity. J Hand Surg Am 1988;13(1):22–8.
9. Godina M. Early microsurgical reconstruction of complex trauma of the extremities. Plast Reconstr Surg 1986;78(3):285–92.
10. Godina M, Bajec J, Baraga A. Salvage of the mutilated upper extremity with temporary ectopic implantation of the undamaged part. Plast Reconstr Surg 1986;78(3):295–9.
11. Chen SH, Wei FC, Chen HC, et al. Emergency free-flap transfer for reconstruction of acute complex extremity wounds. Plast Reconstr Surg 1992;89(5): 882–8 [discussion: 889–90].
12. Sundine M, Scheker LR. A comparison of immediate and staged reconstruction of the dorsum of the hand. J Hand Surg Br 1996;21(2):216–21.
13. Acland RD. Refinements in lower extremity free flap surgery. Clin Plast Surg 1990;17(4):733–44.
14. Grotting JC. Prevention of complications and correction of postoperative problems in microsurgery of the lower extremity. Clin Plast Surg 1991;18(3): 485–9.
15. Kolker AR, Kasabian AK, Karp NS, et al. Fate of free flap microanastomosis distal to the zone of injury in lower extremity trauma. Plast Reconstr Surg 1997; 99(4):1068–73.
16. Bendon CL, Giele HP, Reconstructive Surgery A. Success of free flap anastomoses performed within the zone of trauma in acute lower limb reconstruction. J Plast Reconstr Aesthet Surg 2016;69(7): 888–93.
17. Buncke HJ, Rose EH. Free toe-to-fingertip neurovascular flaps. Plast Reconstr Surg 1979;63(5):607–12.
18. Lee DC, Kim JS, Ki SH, et al. Partial second toe pulp free flap for fingertip reconstruction. Plast Reconstr Surg 2008;121(3):899–907.
19. Tsai TM, Sabapathy SR, Martin D. Revascularization of a finger with a thenar mini-free flap. J Hand Surg Am 1991;16(4):604–6.
20. Kamei K, Ide Y, Kimura T. A new free thenar flap. Plast Reconstr Surg 1993;92(7):1380–4.
21. Sakai S. Free flap from the flexor aspect of the wrist for resurfacing defects of the hand and fingers. Plast Reconstr Surg 2003;111(4):1412–20 [discussion: 21–2].
22. Baek SM. Two new cutaneous free flaps: the medial and lateral thigh flaps. Plast Reconstr Surg 1983; 71(3):354–65.
23. Song YG, Chen GZ, Song YL, et al. The free thigh flap: a new free flap concept based on the septocutaneous artery. Br J Plast Surg 1984;37(2):149–59.
24. Daniel RK, Terzis J, Midgley RD. Restoration of sensation to an anesthetic hand by a free neurovascular flap from the foot. Plast Reconstr Surg 1976; 57(3):275–80.
25. Morrison WA, O'Brien BM, MacLeod AM. Thumb reconstruction with a free neurovascular wrap-around flap from the big toe. J Hand Surg Am 1980;5(6):575–83.
26. Lee HB, Tark KC, Rah DK, et al. Pulp reconstruction of fingers with very small sensate medial plantar free flap. Plast Reconstr Surg 1998;101(4):999–1005.

27. O'brien BM, MacLEOD AM, Hayhurst JW, et al. Successful transfer of a large island flap from the groin to the foot by microvascular anastomoses. Plast Reconstr Surg 1973;52(3):271–8.
28. Morrison WA, O'Brien BM, MacLeod AM, et al. Neurovascular free flaps from the foot for innervation of the hand. J Hand Surg Am 1978;3(3):235–42.
29. Nakayama Y, Soeda S, Kasai YJP, et al. Flaps nourished by arterial inflow through the venous system: an experimental investigation. Plast Reconstr Surg 1981;67(3):328–34.
30. Hauck RM, Camp L, Ehrlich HP, et al. Pulp nonfiction: microscopic anatomy of the digital pulp space. Plast Reconstr Surg 2004;113(2):536–9.
31. Spyropoulou G-A, Shih H-S, Jeng S-F, et al. Free pulp transfer for fingertip reconstruction—the algorithm for complicated Allen fingertip defect. Plast Reconstr Surg Glob Open 2015;3(12):e584.
32. Ratcliffe RJ, McGrouther DA. Free toe pulp transfer in thumb reconstruction. Experience in the West of Scotland Regional Plastic Surgery Unit. J Hand Surg Br 1991;16(2):165–8.
33. Kimura N. Versatility of a second toe plantar flap. J Reconstr Microsurg 2009;25(1):47–53.
34. Cheng G, Fang G, Hou S, et al. Aesthetic reconstruction of thumb or finger partial defect with trimmed toe-flap transfer. Microsurgery 2007;27(2):74–83.
35. Turner A, Ragowannsi R, Hanna J, et al. Microvascular soft tissue reconstruction of the digits. J Plast Reconstr Aesthet Surg 2006;59(5):441–50.
36. Balan JR. Free toe pulp flap for finger pulp and volar defect reconstruction. Indian J Plast Surg 2016;49(2):178–84.
37. Kim HS, Lee DC, Kim JS, et al. Donor-site morbidity after partial second toe pulp free flap for fingertip reconstruction. Arch Plast Surg 2016;43(1):66–70.
38. Yan H, Ouyang Y, Chi Z, et al. Digital pulp reconstruction with free neurovascular toe flaps. Aesthet Plast Surg 2012;36(5):1186–93.
39. Dautel G, Gouzou S, Vialaneix J, et al. PIP reconstruction with vascularized PIP joint from the second toe: minimizing the morbidity with the "dorsal approach and short-pedicle technique. Tech Hand Up Extrem Surg 2004;8(3):173–80.
40. Sun W, Wang Z, Qiu S, et al. Communicating branch of toe web veins as a venous return pathway in free toe pulp flaps. Plast Reconstr Surg 2010;126(5):268e–9e.
41. Sassu P, Lin CH, Lin YT, et al. Fourteen cases of free thenar flap: a rare indication in digital reconstruction. Ann Plast Surg 2008;60(3):260–6.
42. Yang JW, Kim JS, Lee DC, et al. The radial artery superficial palmar branch flap: a modified free thenar flap with constant innervation. J Reconstr Microsurg 2010;26(8):529–38.
43. Chi Z, Pafitanis G, Pont LEP, et al. The use of innervated radial artery superficial palmar branch perforator free flap for complex digital injuries reconstruction. J Plast Surg Hand Surg 2018;52(2):111–6.
44. Lee SH, Cheon SJ, Kim YJ. Clinical application of a free radial artery superficial palmar branch flap for soft-tissue reconstruction of digital injuries. J Hand Surg Eur Vol 2017;42(2):151–6.
45. Zhang GL, Meng H, Huang JH, et al. Reconstruction of digital skin defects with the free wrist crease flap. J Reconstr Microsurg 2015;31(6):471–6.
46. Iwuagwu FC, Orkar SK, Siddiqui A. Reconstruction of volar skin and soft tissue defects of the digits including the pulp: experience with the free SUPBRA flap. J Plast Reconstr Aesthet Surg 2015;68(1):26–34.
47. Lee TP, Liao CY, Wu IC, et al. Free flap from the superficial palmar branch of the radial artery (SPBRA flap) for finger reconstruction. J Trauma 2009;66(4):1173–9.
48. Woo SH, Kim KC, Lee GJ, et al. A retrospective analysis of 154 arterialized venous flaps for hand reconstruction: an 11-year experience. Plast Reconstr Surg 2007;119(6):1823–38.
49. Koshima I, Soeda S, Nakayama Y, et al. An arterialised venous flap using the long saphenous vein. Br J Plast Surg 1991;44(1):23–6.
50. Chen HC, Tang YB, Noordhoff MS. Four types of venous flaps for wound coverage: a clinical appraisal. J Trauma 1991;31(9):1286–93.
51. Inoue G, Tamura YJ. One-stage repair of both skin and tendon digital defects using the arterialized venous flap with palmaris longus tendon. J Reconstr Microsurg 1991;7(04):339–43.
52. Park JU, Kim K, Kwon ST. Venous free flaps for the treatment of skin cancers of the digits. Ann Plast Surg 2015;74(5):536–42.
53. Kayalar M, Kucuk L, Sugun TS, et al. Clinical applications of free arterialized venous flaps. J Plast Reconstr Aesthet Surg 2014;67(11):1548–56.
54. Kong BS, Kim YJ, Suh YS, et al. Finger soft tissue reconstruction using arterialized venous free flaps having 2 parallel veins. J Hand Surg Am 2008;33(10):1802–6.

Soft Tissue Coverage of the Digits and Hand

Soumen Das De, FRCSEd (Ortho), MPH*,
Sandeep J. Sebastin, MCh (Plastic Surgery), MMed (Surgery), FAMS (Hand Surgery)

KEYWORDS

• Soft tissue • Digits • Hand • Reconstruction

KEY POINTS

- There are multiple options available for reconstruction of soft tissue defects of the digits.
- The main goal of reconstruction is to achieve normal or near-normal mobility.
- Soft tissue defects can be considered in the following groups: fingertip, nonfingertip, and multiple digits.
- The choice of reconstruction for fingertip defects depends primarily on the amount of volar skin available.
- The patient's functional demands and expectations, and the expertise of the surgeon, also determine the reconstructive strategy.

INTRODUCTION

Few topics generate as much debate among hand surgeons as soft tissue reconstruction of the hand.[1–5] Soft tissue defects of the digits are one of the commonest problems presenting to orthopedic, plastic, and hand surgeons for specialist care. In the past year, 64 digital defects required reconstruction with flaps at our institution. The flaps that were performed were VY advancement (N = 21), neurovascular island (N = 16), cross-finger (N = 8), reverse vascular island (N = 4), Moberg (N = 3), reverse cross-finger (N = 3), dorsal metacarpal artery perforator (N = 3), heterodigital island (N = 2), free flaps (N = 2), thenar (N = 1) and random design (N = 1). This variety shows the wide spectrum of options available to manage these problems.

There is no such thing as the ideal flap, and a specific defect can be addressed with a variety of flaps with similar outcomes. There are choices that cater to surgeons of all levels of expertise and proficiency. The difficulty often faced by surgeons is choosing the right flap for the right patient. The literature is replete with case series presenting the experience of a single author or institution, but there are few comparative studies that clearly show the superiority of any particular option. This article presents a simple approach to evaluating soft tissue defects of the hand and highlights the goals of soft tissue reconstruction to provide a basis for rational decision making in choosing an appropriate flap, and a few tips and technical nuances are suggested for individual flaps to improve outcomes.

GENERAL APPROACH TO DIGITAL DEFECTS

As discussed earlier, there is a wide variety of reconstructive options with scant evidence supporting one flap rather than another. It is important to choose the most straightforward option that addresses all the reconstructive needs while minimizing donor site morbidity. The various flaps can be classified based on contiguity to the defect: homodigital, heterodigital, local (hand), regional (forearm), distant (groin/cross-arm), and free flaps. Homodigital flaps are further categorized into

Department of Hand & Reconstructive Microsurgery, National University Health System, Tower Block, Level 11, 1E Kent Ridge Road, Singapore 119228
* Corresponding author.
E-mail address: das_de_soumen@nuhs.edu.sg

Hand Clin 36 (2020) 97–105
https://doi.org/10.1016/j.hcl.2019.09.002

random-pattern, axial-pattern, or perforator-based flaps, depending on the pattern of vascularization. **Box 1** lists the important factors when deciding on the most appropriate form of reconstruction. Another consideration is the level of technical difficulty. This article divided flaps into easy, moderate, and hard. Easy flaps do not require vascular dissection and should be frontline choices for surgeons in training. Flaps of moderate difficulty require vascular dissection, whereas the technically difficult flaps require microsurgical expertise and resources.

Important considerations during digital flap reconstruction include:

1. Use a thin flap. The primary goal of soft tissue reconstruction in the hand is to ensure that the reconstructed digit regains normal or near-normal motion. This goal requires thin and pliable skin that allows digital flexion and gliding of the underlying tendons. Skin grafts adhere to the underlying soft tissue and can limit motion, especially where they cross joints, whereas a bulky flap is a physical block to digital flexion. If an adipofascial flap is being considered, it is preferable to use a full-thickness skin graft rather than a split-thickness skin graft because the former is more durable and can resist secondary contracture better.
2. Design flaps from injured digit as much as possible. In general, the authors prefer not to use an uninjured digit for reconstruction of digital defects. Although the adjacent digits are a readily available source of similar tissue, the inevitable scarring that results will hamper motion of the donor finger. In addition, issues such as hypersensitivity and paresthesia can significantly affect global hand function. Our preference is to use tissue from the same finger, if possible, or from the hand. If a heterodigital flap is necessary, we usually take it as an adipofascial flap and resurface both the flap and the donor defect with a full-thickness skin graft.
3. Use flaps for resurfacing critical defects only. During the initial assessment, the surgeon should divide the defect into critical and noncritical areas. Noncritical areas are those portions that are amenable to linear closure and/or skin grafting. Critical areas involve exposed bone, joint, tendon, and/or neurovascular structures and usually require a flap. Making this distinction allows a smaller flap to be used to cover the important areas and reduces donor site morbidity (**Fig. 1**).
4. Single-stage reconstruction. Defects in the hand often involve multiple tissues and may require concomitant repair or reconstruction of bone, joint, tendon, and the nail complex. It is preferable to address these injuries in a single stage unless contraindicated for specific reasons; for example, staged flexor tendon reconstruction in the setting of extensive damage to the pulleys. The surgeon must decide whether each damaged tissue component should be reconstructed individually with grafts or whether the additional tissues should be incorporated within the flap (ie, a composite flap). For example, a heterodigital flap can be used for digit revascularization using a flow-through design while simultaneously achieving soft tissue coverage.

Box 1
Considerations in digital and hand soft tissue reconstruction

Defect characteristics

- Location (fingertip vs nonfingertip)
- Level of amputation
- Geometry
- Size
- Number of digits involved (adjacent vs nonadjacent)

Technical considerations

- Level of difficulty
- Available resources

Patient factors

- Hand dominance
- Occupation and functional demands
- Preexisting illnesses; for example, diabetes, peripheral vascular disease, renal impairment
- Compliance with postoperative rehabilitation plan
- Cosmetic concerns, preferences, and expectations

Soft tissue reconstruction is discussed here in the following areas: (1) fingertip defects, (2) nonfingertip defects, and (3) multiple nonfingertip defects.

Fingertip Defects

The fingertip comprises the nail complex, specialized pulp, distal interphalangeal joint (DIPJ), and the flexor and extensor tendon insertions. There are many algorithms that deal with fingertip amputations and they usually focus on the level of the amputation and geometry of the resultant defect.[6,7]

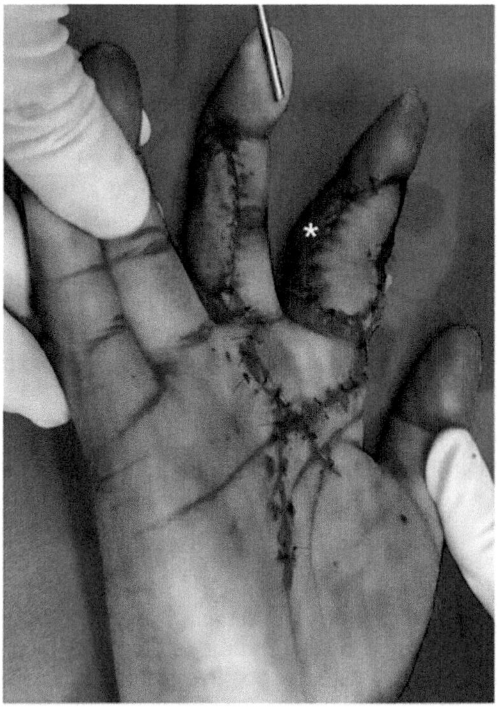

Fig. 1. Critical and noncritical defects. A heterodigital vascular island flap from the middle finger was used to resurface an index finger soft tissue defect. The flap was designed to cover the flexor tendon and adjacent neurovascular bundles, whereas the dorsal aspect of the defect was resurfaced using a full-thickness skin graft from the medial forearm (*asterisk*).

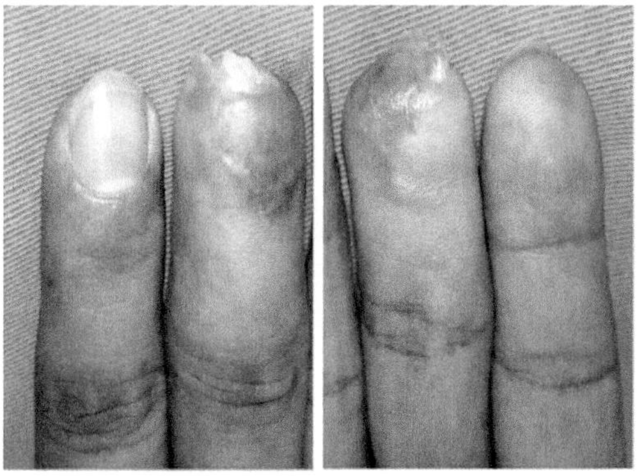

Fig. 2. Fingertip amputations with inadequate remaining nail. Amputation proximal to the level of the lunula resulted in a very small amount of remaining nail complex. The nail was retained and a skin graft was used to resurface the volar skin defect. The resulting nail has no bony support, is irregular, and does not have a smooth cuticle layer. The fingertip is unsightly and the nail tends to catch on clothing. A better option would have been amputation through the DIPJ.

1. Level of amputation. The level of amputation determines the need for flap reconstruction. There is a paucity of evidence that shows a functional benefit of fingertip reconstruction rather than amputation.[1,8,9] In our opinion, fingertip reconstruction is an aesthetic procedure and should only be considered when a reasonable-looking fingertip can be reconstructed. The minimum requirement for this is the presence of a useful nail (**Fig. 2**). We therefore consider fingertip reconstruction for amputations at or distal to the lunula. For situations in which only 1 to 2 mm of visible nail matrix is available, an eponychial recession flap can be performed to increase the amount of visible nail.[10,11] If there is less than this amount of nail left, we recommend a terminalization through the DIPJ rather than through the base of the distal phalanx because the proximal end of the nail bed is just 1 and 2 mm distal to the flexor and extensor tendon insertions, respectively. A terminalization that requires no nail bed remnants requires the dorsal skin to be incised at or immediately distal to the DIPJ crease. An amputation that attempts to preserve the tendon insertions and good soft tissue cover therefore leaves a very short stump of bone and the DIPJ will usually not move because of the limited moment arm.In summary, the decision to proceed with flap reconstruction for fingertip amputations is based on the amount of remaining nail bed, and reconstruction is reserved for patients with amputations at or distal to the lunula.
2. Geometry of the defect. The geometry of the defect determines the type of flap that is required. Previous classifications have used terms such as volar unfavorable, transverse, oblique, and so forth to describe the geometry of the defect. The authors think that it is not the geometry of the defect but the amount of pulp skin remaining after debridement that determines the type of flap required (**Fig. 3**). The adult fingertip (thumb tip) is on an average 25 to 30 mm long (from DIPJ crease to the hyponychium). If greater than or equal to 20 mm of pulp skin is available, a VY advancement flap can be considered. If there is 15 to 20 mm of pulp skin available, a homodigital neurovascular island (NVI) flap (Moberg for thumb) can be considered, and if less than or equal to 15 mm of pulp skin is available, a reverse vascular island (RVI) flap (cross-finger flap, heterodigital NVI, or a toe pulp transfer for thumb) is preferred.

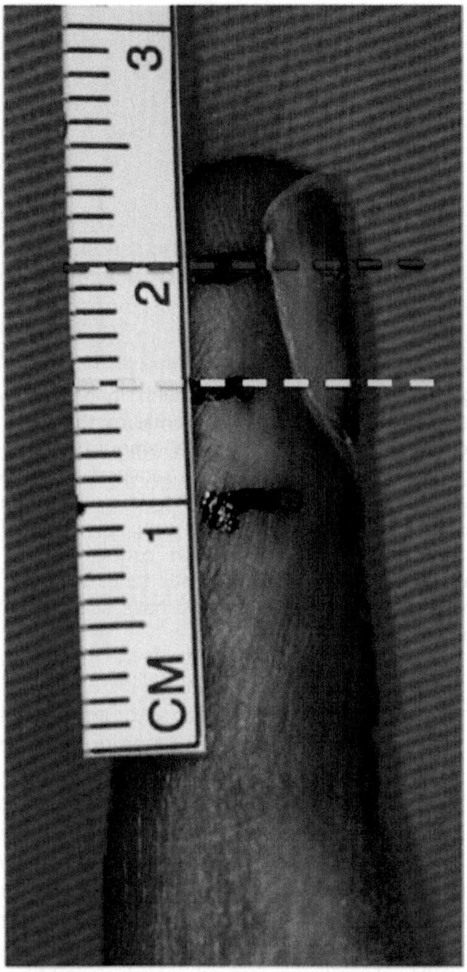

Fig. 3. Decision making in fingertip defects. In amputations with 2 cm or more of pulp skin remaining (*red dashed line*), a VY advancement flap achieves good coverage. If there is 1.5 to 2 cm of skin available (*yellow dashed line*), a homodigital neurovascular island (NVI) flap is preferred. In defects with less than 1.5 cm of available skin, a reverse vascular island (RVI) flap is used.

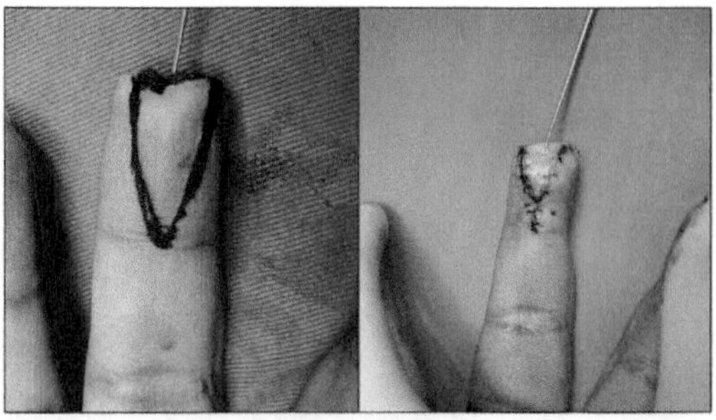

Fig. 4. VY advancement flap. A champagne-glass technique allows the lateral nailfolds to be elegantly reconstructed without leaving unsightly overhanging folds. Adequate mobilization of the flap is achieved by incising the skin completely at the apex of the flap (at the distal interphalangeal crease) and the distal 5 mm of skin.

This approach assists surgeons in selecting the simplest homodigital option that provides an aesthetically pleasing and painless fingertip. The common flaps used for fingertip defects are discussed next.

VY advancement flap

Tranquilli-Leali and Atasoy described 2 slightly different versions of the VY advancement flap.[12] Approximately 4 to 6 mm of advancement can be achieved by incising the skin completely at the apex of the flap (at the distal interphalangeal crease) and the distal 5 mm of skin (**Fig. 4**). In the intervening areas, the subcutaneous septae are released with a blade using gentle pressure. The flap should be completely dissected free from the underlying periosteum and flexor sheath. The flap is advanced and the distal nailfold is sutured first. If the flap appears pale after releasing the tourniquet, the proximal sutures should be released and any resulting defects may be covered with small skin grafts. The main problem is inadequate release of the underlying septa, resulting in a flattened pulp and a hook-nail deformity.

Neurovascular island flap

Segmuller[13] reported on a modification of the Kutler flap in which the neurovascular bundle is mobilized to increase excursion of the flap. Venkataswami and Subramanian[14] subsequently described the oblique triangular flap for coverage of oblique fingertip amputations. The homodigital NVI flap that we use takes elements of both concepts (**Fig. 5**). Our own cadaveric studies indicate that an average advancement of about 12 mm can be achieved if the neurovascular bundle is dissected up to the palmodigital crease (unpublished data). A generous cuff of tissue is left around the neurovascular bundle to avoid damage to the venae comitantes that spiral around the digital artery.

Reverse vascular island flap

There are several retrotendinous, transverse anastomoses between the radial and ulnar digital arteries. The RVI is perfused via the middle transverse palmar arch, which passes deep to the flexor tendon at the level of middle phalangeal neck.[15] The flap can be used to resurface defects involving the entire pulp as well as dorsal digital defects (**Fig. 6**). The authors recommend

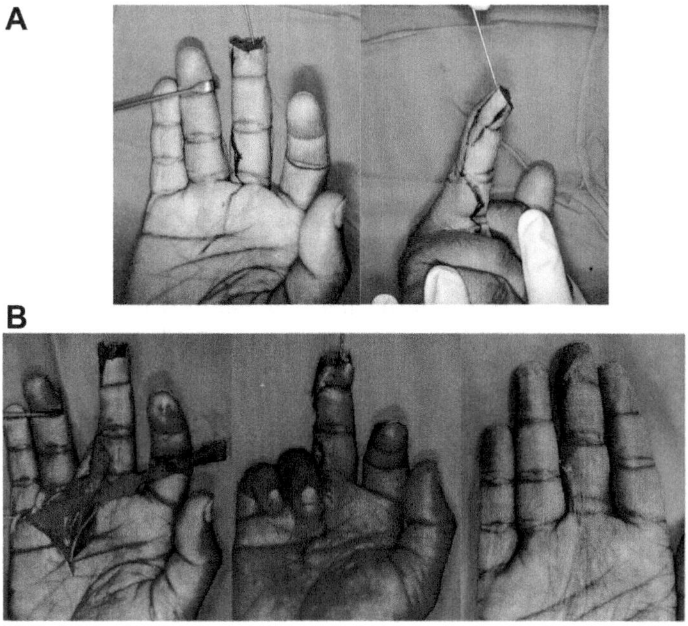

Fig. 5. NVI flap. (*A*) The flap is designed along the lateral aspect of the digit. The blind (ulnar) side is selected for the index and middle fingers. A zigzag incision proximally allows tension-free closure. The web space must be avoided as the incision is carried into the palm in order to prevent contractures. (*B*) The flap is advanced along the lateral border of the digit to achieve a well-contoured pulp. Skin grafts should be used over noncritical areas and proximal interphalangeal joint mobilization exercises are initiated within 2 to 3 days after surgery.

cutting directly on the nerve sheath with a blade using gentle pressure and retracting it away from the digital artery using a vessel loop; this ensures that the venae comitantes remain undisturbed. Subdermal dissection at the edges of the flap makes the flap less bulky.

Nonfingertip Defects

The choice of flaps for reconstruction of nonfingertip defects is primarily determined by the size of the defect. A good way to quantify size is to think of 1 surface (palmar or dorsal) of a phalangeal segment (proximal phalanx, middle phalanx, or distal phalanx) as 1 unit (**Fig. 7**). A small defect involves 1 unit, a medium-sized defect involves 2 contiguous units, and a large defect involves 3 or more contiguous units or 2 noncontiguous units. Small defects are typically less than 4 cm^2; medium-sized defects 4 to 8 cm^2, and large defects are usually greater than 8 cm^2.

Table 1 lists the various options for nonfingertip defects. Our preferred options for small nonfingertip defects are adipofascial turndown and digital artery perforator flaps.[16] Alternative options are the cross-finger and reverse dermis cross-finger flaps. For the thumb, small nonpulp defects can be resurfaced using a Brunelli flap.[17] Medium-sized defects can be resurfaced using a dorsal metacarpal artery (DMA) perforator flap[18] for the fingers and the first dorsal metacarpal artery (FDMA) flap[19] for the thumb. Suitable alternatives are the heterodigital adipofascial vascular island flap, cross-finger flap, or small free flaps. Large defects are ideally addressed using pedicled flaps from the forearm.

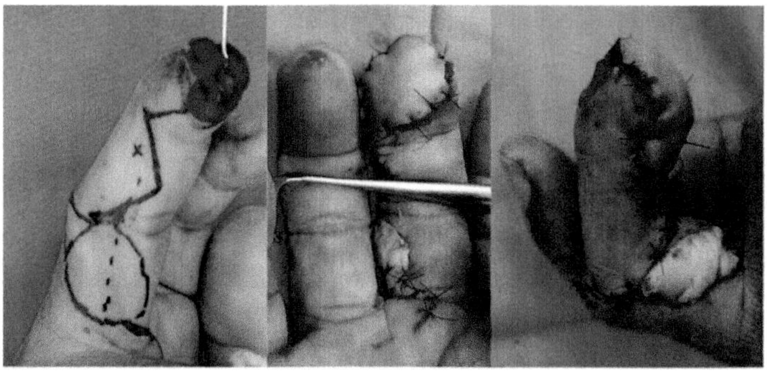

Fig. 6. RVI flap. The RVI flap is designed with a tail arising from the lax dorsal skin. The resultant dorsal defect can be closed primarily and the tail comes to lie over the pedicle. The pivot point of the flap (marked x) is the point where the retrotendinous transverse arch emerges to join the ulnar and radial digital arteries.

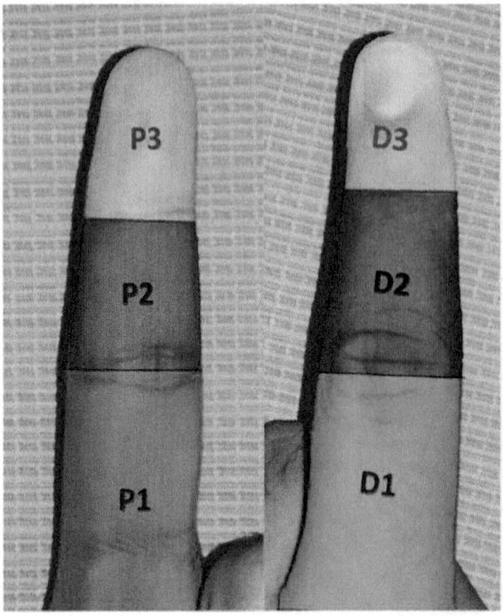

Fig. 7. Nonfingertip defects. Nonfingertip defects can be classified as small, medium, or large defects depending on the number of units involved. A unit comprises 1 surface, either palmar (P) or dorsal (D), of a single phalangeal segment.

Dorsal metacarpal artery flap

Quaba and Davison[18] described a dorsal hand flap based on perforators from the dorsal metacarpal artery or dorsal perforators from the deep palmar arch or palmar metacarpal arteries. The cutaneous perforators of the DMA arise at the level of the metacarpal neck in the second to fourth intermetacarpal spaces, just distal to the juncture tendinae. The skin over the dorsum of the hand is thin and pliable, and provides an excellent match for resurfacing dorsal hand and finger defects.[20] The donor defect can be closed linearly in most cases. It is preferable to do the initial debridement under wrist/brachial blocks (instead of a digital block) to preserve the dorsal perforators and accompanying veins around the metacarpal neck. This flap can reliably resurface defects up to the proximal third of the middle phalanx. The use of a curved elliptical flap design can allow more distal reach when the flap is rotated and straightened. We exclude any large cutaneous veins traversing the edge of the flap. They do not help with venous drainage and increase the risk of congestion. In addition, this is a low flow flap and clinicians should avoid tunneling the flap under an intact skin bridge.

First dorsal metacarpal artery flap

The FDMA arises from the deep branch of the radial artery before it dives between the heads of the first dorsal interosseous muscle to enter the palm. The FDMA reliably perfuses the dorsal skin up to the middle of the proximal phalanx of the index finger. The skin circulation becomes random and the flap is less reliable beyond this point. The flap may be raised as an island or with a tail of skin from the dorsum of the first web space.[19] It is important that the FDMA is retained in a broad strip of fascia and not skeletonized during flap elevation (**Fig. 8**). A broad tunnel in the first web space

Table 1
Flaps for nonfingertip digital defects

Small Defects (1 Unit)	Medium Defects (2 Units)	Large Defects (>2 Units)
Homodigital (preferred) • Adipofascial[a] • Digital artery perforator[b] • Brunelli (thumb)[a] Heterodigital • Cross-finger flap[a] • Heterodigital (neuro) vascular island[b]	Hand (preferred) • Dorsal metacarpal artery perforator[a] • First dorsal metacarpal artery (thumb)[a] Heterodigital • Cross-finger flap[a] • Heterodigital (neuro) vascular island/adipofascial[b] Free • Ulnar artery perforator[c] • Radial artery perforator[c] • Superficial radial artery[c]	Regional • Radial forearm[b] • Posterior interosseous artery (thumb)[b] Distant • Groin/abdomen[a] • Lateral arm[a] Free • Radial forearm[c]

[a] Easy.
[b] Moderate.
[c] Difficult.

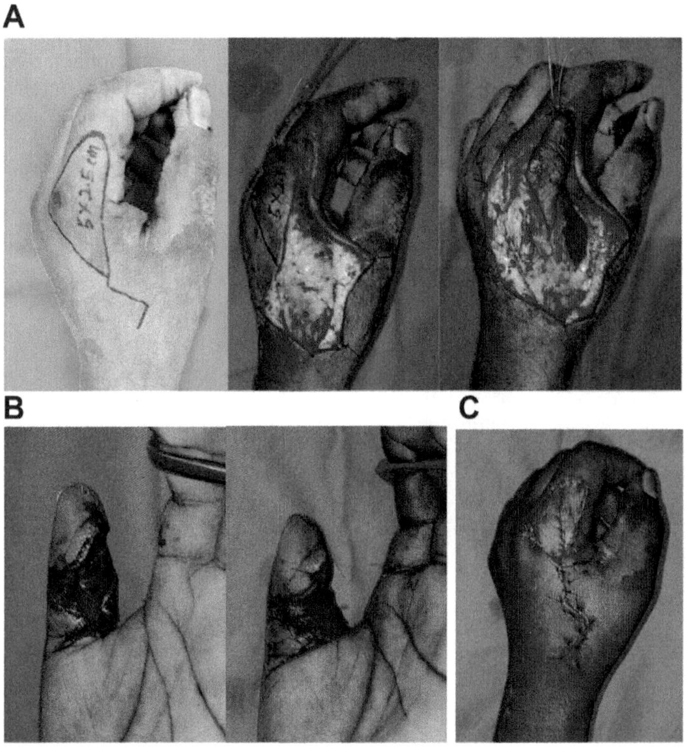

Fig. 8. FDMA flap. (*A*) The flap is designed over the index metacarpophalangeal joint and up to the middle of the proximal phalanx (*left*). The fascia over the first dorsal interosseous muscle is incised and a broad strip of fascia is taken (*middle and right*). (*B*) Thumb defect before (*left*) and after (*right*) reconstruction with an FDMA flap. (*C*) A full-thickness skin graft from the medial forearm was used to resurface the donor site defect. A posterior interosseous nerve graft was also used to reconstruct a segmental defect of the ulnar digital nerve.

must be made to avoid compression on the pedicle.

Defects Involving Multiple Digits

The reconstructive needs differ greatly depending on the number of digits involved. In the setting of multiple digit involvement, surgeons must consider whether these are adjacent or nonadjacent digits. Adjacent digits allow the creation of a temporary syndactyly, thus converting multiple defects into a single defect. We prefer to use a pedicled radial forearm flap for multiple adjacent digits. Other options include abdominal/groin flaps or thin free flaps such as the radial forearm flap. A division of the syndactyly is performed at a later stage (**Fig. 9**). Severe mangling injuries of the hand may render reconstruction of some digits a futile attempt. In these situations, amputating the severely damaged digit and using its components for soft tissue coverage (eg, a heterodigital island flap) or for spare parts to address bone, tendon, and nerve defects is a good solution.

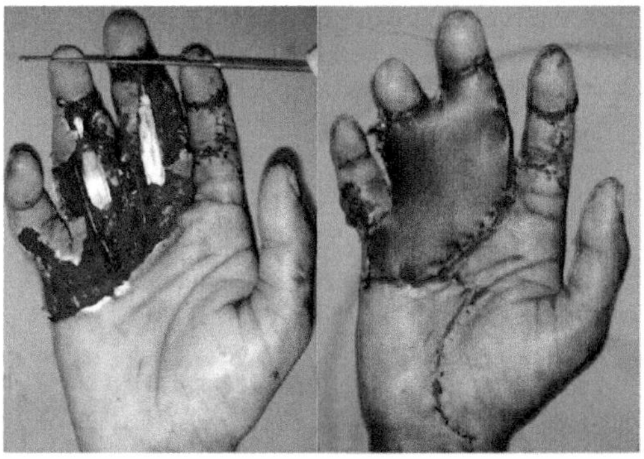

Fig. 9. Multiple digital defects (adjacent digits). Large defects of 3 adjacent digits (*left*) were resurfaced using a pedicle radial forearm flap. The digits were syndactylized (*right*) and were separated in staged fashion.

For multiple nonadjacent digits, using a single flap unnecessarily immobilizes the uninvolved digits. It is best to consider each digital defect on its own and determine whether a simple solution (eg, skin grafts, homodigital flaps) will work. If the defects are all of moderate size, multiple random-pattern abdominal (Louvre) flaps are a good option[21] (**Fig. 10**). The inconvenience of having the hand immobilized for a period of 2 to 3 weeks is offset by the abundant source of tissue and a concealed donor site. The flaps may be thinned at the time of flap division.

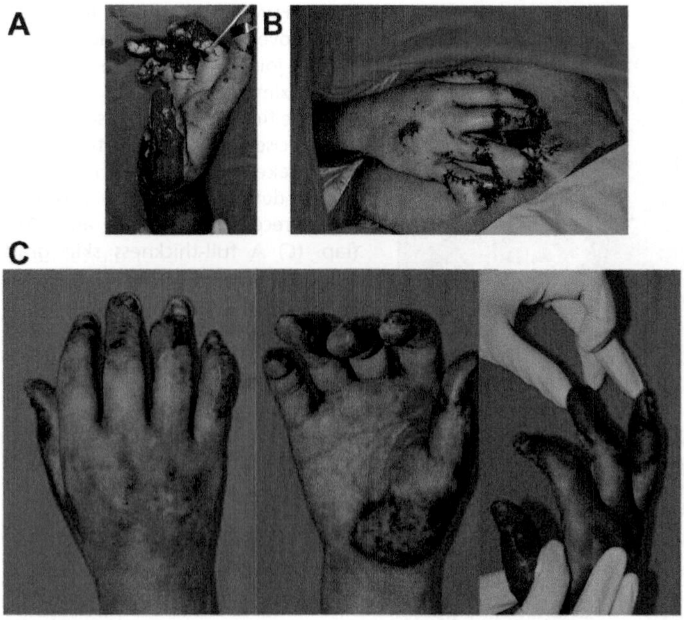

Fig. 10. Multiple digital defects (nonadjacent digits). (*A*) Multiple defects involving several nonadjacent digits. (*B*) Multiple random-pattern abdominal (Louvre) flaps were used to resurface the defects. (*C*) Postoperative outcome.

SUMMARY

There are multiple options available for reconstruction of soft tissue defects of the digits. The main goal of reconstruction is to achieve normal or near-normal mobility. Soft tissue defects can be considered in the following groups: fingertip, nonfingertip, and multiple digits. The choice of reconstruction for fingertip defects depends primarily on the amount of volar skin available. Nonfingertip defects can be considered as small, medium, or large depending on the number of units involved. In addition, the choice of reconstruction for multiple digit injuries depends on whether the digits are adjacent to each other or nonadjacent. The patient's functional demands and expectations, and the expertise of the surgeon, also determine the reconstructive strategy.

DISCLOSURE

The authors have nothing to disclose.

REFERENCES

1. Miller AJ, Rivlin M, Kirkpatrick W, et al. Fingertip amputation treatment: a survey study. Am J Orthop (Belle Mead NJ) 2015;44(9):E331–9.
2. Bickel KD, Dosanjh A. Fingertip reconstruction. J Hand Surg Am 2008;33(8):1417–9.
3. Hart RG, Kleinert HE. Fingertip and nail bed injuries. Emerg Med Clin North Am 1993;11(3):755–65.
4. Martin C, Gonzalez del Pino J. Controversies in the treatment of fingertip amputations. conservative versus surgical reconstruction. Clin Orthop Relat Res 1998;353(353):63–73.
5. Soderberg T, Nystrom A, Hallmans G, et al. Treatment of fingertip amputations with bone exposure. A comparative study between surgical and conservative treatment methods. Scand J Plast Reconstr Surg 1983;17(2):147–52.
6. Lemmon JA, Janis JE, Rohrich RJ. Soft-tissue injuries of the fingertip: methods of evaluation and treatment. an algorithmic approach. Plast Reconstr Surg 2008;122(3):105e–17e.
7. Tang JB, Elliot D, Adani R, et al. Repair and reconstruction of thumb and finger tip injuries: a global view. Clin Plast Surg 2014;41(3):325–59.
8. van den Berg WB, Vergeer RA, van der Sluis CK, et al. Comparison of three types of treatment modalities on the outcome of fingertip injuries. J Trauma Acute Care Surg 2012;72(6):1681–7.
9. Weichman KE, Wilson SC, Samra F, et al. Treatment and outcomes of fingertip injuries at a large metropolitan public hospital. Plast Reconstr Surg 2013;131(1):107–12.
10. Adani R, Marcoccio I, Tarallo L. Nail lengthening and fingertip amputations. Plast Reconstr Surg 2003;112(5):1287–94.
11. Adani R, Leo G, Tarallo L. Nail salvage using the eponychial flap. Tech Hand Up Extrem Surg 2006;10(4):255–8.
12. Gharb BB, Rampazzo A, Armijo BS, et al. Tranquilli-leali or atasoy flap: an anatomical cadaveric study. J Plast Reconstr Aesthet Surg 2010;63(4):681–5.
13. Segmuller G. Modification of the kutler flap: neurovascular pedicle. Handchirurgie 1976;8(2):75–6.

14. Venkataswami R, Subramanian N. Oblique triangular flap: a new method of repair for oblique amputations of the fingertip and thumb. Plast Reconstr Surg 1980;66(2):296–300.
15. Adani R, Busa R, Pancaldi G, et al. Reverse neurovascular homodigital island flap. Ann Plast Surg 1995;35(1):77–82.
16. Koshima I, Urushibara K, Fukuda N, et al. Digital artery perforator flaps for fingertip reconstructions. Plast Reconstr Surg 2006;118(7):1579–84.
17. Brunelli F, Vigasio A, Valenti P, et al. Arterial anatomy and clinical application of the dorsoulnar flap of the thumb. J Hand Surg Am 1999;24(4):803–11.
18. Quaba AA, Davison PM. The distally-based dorsal hand flap. Br J Plast Surg 1990;43(1):28–39.
19. Foucher G, Braun JB. A new island flap transfer from the dorsum of the index to the thumb. Plast Reconstr Surg 1979;63(3):344–9.
20. Sebastin SJ, Mendoza RT, Chong AK, et al. Application of the dorsal metacarpal artery perforator flap for resurfacing soft-tissue defects proximal to the fingertip. Plast Reconstr Surg 2011;128(3):166e–78e.
21. Emmett AJ. Finger resurfacing by the multiple subcutaneous pedicle or louvre flaps. Br J Plast Surg 1974;27(4):370–4.

A Review and Meta-analysis of Adverse Events Related to Local Flap Reconstruction for Digital Soft Tissue Defects

Teemu Karjalainen, MD, PhD[a,b,*], Jarkko Jokihaara, MD, PhD[c,d]

KEYWORDS

• Adverse event • Complication • Hand • Surgical flaps • Systematic review • Meta-analysis

KEY POINTS

- Choose the flap primarily based on functional requirements of the patient and defect site as well as the surgeon's personal preferences because the risk of adverse events is acceptable in all flaps.
- Reverse flow flaps and digital artery perforator-based flaps may be at higher risk for vascular insufficiency (partial or total loss of flap) compared with flaps with antegrade flow or skin pedicle.
- Patients undergoing pedicled flap reconstruction can be informed that risk for adverse event is likely between 1% and 10% (average 5.4%) depending on the flap type; reoperations are needed in approximately 2% of cases.

INTRODUCTION

Local pedicled flaps are reliable options to cover digital soft tissue defects typically caused by trauma. Although these flaps usually do not require actual microsurgery, the surgeon needs to be competent in tissue handling and be familiar with the intricate anatomy of the hand. Sometimes surgeons make poor decisions in flap design or encounters technical difficulties, and this may result in loss of flap. Poor choice or design of the flap may also impair hand function as the flap may be too bulky; the fingertip may be rendered scarred, insensate, or hypersensitive; and there may be scar contractures, or donor site complications.

All adverse events encountered after flap reconstruction should not be attributed to the flap surgery itself. The trauma causing the defect often destroys the intricate anatomic structures and normal function is often impossible to restore. For example, fingertips are densely innervated and injury may result in chronic pain regardless of the flap; excessive contamination may cause infection despite meticulous debridement; and trauma to the tendons and joints may result in loss of motion even in the absence of any associated soft tissue defects.

Recognizing the potential problems helps to choose the flap with least risks. Knowing the typical

Disclosure Statement: T. Karjalainen has received funding from Finnish Medical Association and Finnish Centre for evidence Based Medicine (FICEBO). The funding sources have no role in the gathering, analysis, interpretation of the data, or preparing or writing this article.

[a] Department of Epidemiology and Preventive Medicine, School of Public Health and Preventive Medicine, Monash Department of Clinical Epidemiology, Cabrini Hospital, Monash University, Malvern, Australia; [b] Department of Surgery, Central Finland Central Hospital, Keskussairaalantie 16, Jyväskylä 40620, Finland; [c] Department of Hand Surgery, Tampere University Hospital, TAYS/TUL2, Teiskontie 35, Tampere 33521, Finland; [d] Faculty of Medicine and Health Technology, Tampere University, TAYS/TUL2, Teiskontie 35, Tampere 33521, Finland
* Corresponding author. Keskussairaalantie 16, Jyväskylä 40620, Finland.
E-mail address: teemukarjalainen@me.com

Hand Clin 36 (2020) 107–121
https://doi.org/10.1016/j.hcl.2019.08.009

pitfalls for each flap also helps paying attention to crucial technical aspects. Furthermore, the patient can be informed about the expected outcome and risks before surgery. Myriad of studies report outcomes after different flap reconstructions, but we were not able to identify systematic reviews to inform stakeholders about the incidence of adverse events. Thus, our objective was to review the current literature to identify studies reporting flap reconstructions, and to perform a meta-analysis to estimate the incidence of adverse events for different type of local pedicled flaps of the hand.

METHODS

Search Strategy

We conducted a search in MEDLINE, Embase, and CENTRAL databases from their inception to December 1, 2018. We searched using the following terms: (hand OR thumb OR phalangeal OR thenar OR palm) AND (skin flap OR pedicled skin flap OR island flap OR neurovascular island flap OR digital flap OR phalangeal flap OR heterodigital flap OR homodigital flap OR venous flap OR thenar flap OR cross finger OR CFF OR adipofascial flap OR fasciosubcutaneous flap OR metacarpal artery flap OR perforator flap OR turnover flap OR reverse ADJ3 flap OR kite flap OR VY-plasty OR Moberg flap OR Hueston flap).

Eligibility

We formulated the research question using the PICO format (**Table 1**). We accepted any study design as long as it included at least 5 participants and reported the number of vascular complications (partial or complete loss of flap as reported by the investigators). If the article did not mention the vascular complications and we could not determine complications from the data (eg, tables), we excluded the paper. When the same investigator had published 2 articles of same flap within an overlapping period, we excluded the smaller series. We also excluded studies that reported outcomes for a subset of a cohort and did not report the vascular complications for the whole cohort; if the flaps were used to cover defects outside hand; if greater than 10% of the flaps were covered to correct deformities (eg, congenital or nail); if the article reported several flaps and we could not extract the adverse events for each flap type; or if flaps required microvascular anastomosis (arterial of venous).

Table 1
The PICO chart for the review

*P*roblem	Soft tissue defect of the hand (distal to wrist)
*I*ntervention	Local pedicled flap raised from hand
*C*ontrol	Any or no control
*O*utcome	Proportion of patients suffering adverse event as defined by the authors

Study Selection, Data Extraction, and Handling

One author screened the titles and abstracts to identify potentially eligible studies. If the studies were written in a language other than English, we translated the article or a native speaker extracted the data. One author assessed the full texts of potentially eligible studies, if there was doubt, the other author was consulted. One author extracted the study characteristics and numbers for adverse events, and the other author checked the data.

We categorized the flaps to the following categories: cross finger flaps (CFF); dorsal metacarpal artery flaps (DMCA, including also DMCA perforator-based, and extended DMCA flaps); dorsal adipofascial flaps; neurovascular island flaps (NVI; homodigital or heterodigital); digital artery perforator flaps (including flaps based on dorsal connections of thumb digital arteries); random transposition flaps; reverse vascular island flaps (RVI); thenar flaps; venous flaps; volar palmar artery–based flaps; or VY-plasty. We then calculated the rates for different adverse events as sum of adverse events for each flap type divided by the total number of each flap. We report all the estimates with 95% confidence intervals (CI).

We categorized the complication as vascular (total or partial loss of flap) and nonvascular (bulky flap, inadequate cover, scar contracture, infection, bleeding requiring procedure, donor site problem requiring secondary intervention, pain related such as neuroma or chronic regional pain syndrome). We planned to include severe cold intolerance, but cold intolerance was reported so heterogeneously that the reliable rates of could not usually be extracted. Regarding pain-related adverse events, we recorded cases in which the participants were reported to have a painful neuroma, severe hyperesthesia, or complex regional pain syndrome. We recorded other complications as the authors had defined. We considered nail deformities to be trauma related and did not consider them as adverse events in this review.

RESULTS

The results of the search are shown in **Fig. 1**. We included 241 cohort studies (some reported

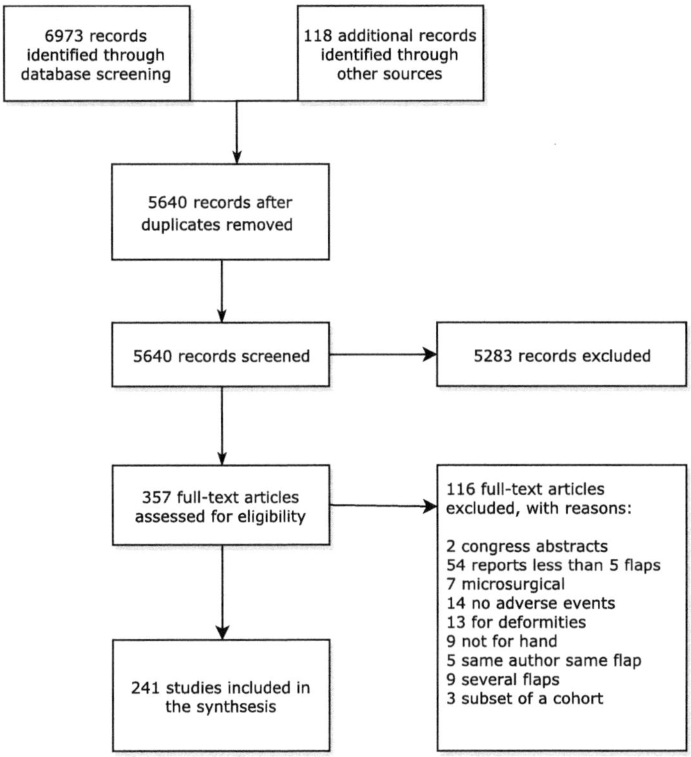

Fig. 1. Flowchart of the study.

more than 1 type of flap) published between 1965 and 2018, which reported the number of vascular complications in 6693 flaps performed for 6167 patients. Thirty-one studies included 976 CFFs,[1–31] 54 studies included 1096 DMCA-based flaps,[32–86] 12 studies included 204 dorsal adipofascial transposition flaps,[24,87–97] 52 studies included 1682 direct flow NVI flaps,[5,17,98–146] 31 studies included 820 digital artery perforator-based flaps,[77,81,83,147–175] 9 studies included 216 random transposition flaps,[98,176–183] 33 studies included 846 RVI flaps,[5,137,184–214] 9 studies included 262 thenar flaps,[215–224] 2 studies reported 33 venous flaps,[225,226] 9 studies included 105 volar palmar artery–based flaps,[227–235] and 6 studies included 456 VY-plasties.[5,17,236–239] (**Table 2**).

Most of the studies also reported other complications or lack of them. We identified 1 randomized controlled trial (RCT) comparing reverse and direct flow digital flaps but it did not report adverse events and was thus excluded from the analysis.[240] We did not identify any registries designed for recording adverse events systematically. After full-text review, we excluded 116 studies (see **Fig. 1**), most often (n = 54 studies, 47% of excluded) due to reporting only the technique or a cohort of fewer than 5 patients.

The defects were dominantly caused by trauma (95%) and occurred typically in thumb, index, or long finger, each comprising a quarter of the total number of injured digits. The ulnar digits or hand were affected less frequently (**Table 3**).

The rate of any adverse event was 5.4% (n = 359 of all 6693 flaps). The most common reported adverse event was vascular complication (partial or complete loss of flap), which occurred in 3.3% (n = 225) of all 6719 flaps.

Partial loss was more common compared with total loss occurring in 2.7% (n = 182) and 0.6% (n = 43) of flaps, respectively. The highest rates of vascular compromise were reported in venous flaps, proper digital artery perforator-based flaps, DMCA-based flaps, and RVI flaps (**Fig. 2**). Because the vascular complications carried the most weight in the meta-analysis, the same flaps that had highest rates of vascular adverse events also had the highest rates of all complications (see **Fig. 2**).

Nonvascular adverse events were generally less frequent (<2%) when cold intolerance was not included (see **Fig. 2**, **Table 4**). The incidence of cold intolerance was reported so heterogeneously that we decided not to pool the data.

Table 2
The number of flap types and participants

Flap	Flaps, n	Studies, n	Participants, n	Male, %[a]	Gender Missing, %[a]
CFF	976	31	942	74	42
DMCA	1096	54	1027	77	14
Dorsal adipofascial	204	12	200	91	22
NVI	1682	52	1518	84	41
Digital perforator	820	31	675	78	7
Random transposition	216	9	147	77	42
RVI	846	33	791	81	13
Thenar	262	9	253	79	23
Venous	33	2	30	100	80
Volar palmar artery	105	9	105	72	29
VY-plasty	456	6	456	79	91
TOTAL	6693	241[b]	6167	81	32

Abbreviations: CFF, cross finger flap; DMCA, dorsal metacarpal artery–based flap; NVI, neurovascular island flap; RVI, reverse vascular island flap.

[a] Proportion of male individuals is calculated from the studies that report sex. Proportion of missing values calculated from total number of flaps.

[b] Total number of different studies (some studies reported several type of flaps).

Some studies reported all participants had some cold intolerance, whereas most reports did not comment at all or declared no "serious" cold intolerance. Rate of reoperation related to original flap reconstruction (excluding reoperations for other reasons such as nonunion or tendon adhesions) was 1.9% (n = 126 reoperations with 6693 flaps) (**Fig. 3**).

Table 3
The location of recipient sites by flap type

Flap	Flaps, n	Hand, %[a]	Thumb, %[a]	Index, %[a]	Middle, %[a]	Ring, %[a]	Little, %[a]	Missing, %[b]
CFF	976	0	42	20	18	12	8	57
DMCA	1096	8	36	27	17	9	5	11
Dorsal adipofascial	204	12	17	19	22	21	10	5
NVI	1682	3	38	24	20	11	4	52
Digital perforator	820	0	18	27	29	18	8	6
Random transposition	216	0	10	30	26	19	14	28
RVI	846	0	1	35	34	21	9	23
Thenar	262	0	0	42	36	19	2	65
Venous	33	0	0	0	43	29	29	79
Volar palmar artery	105	11	13	22	18	11	24	53
VY-plasty	456	0	39	36	25	0	0	91
TOTAL	6693	3	25	27	24	15	7	38

Due to rounding, the percentages do not always add up to 100.

Abbreviations: CFF, cross finger flap; DMCA, dorsal metacarpal artery–based flap; NVI, neurovascular island flap; RVI, reverse vascular island flap.

[a] Proportions for each finger calculated from the studies reporting that detail.

[b] Proportion of missing values calculated from total number of flaps.

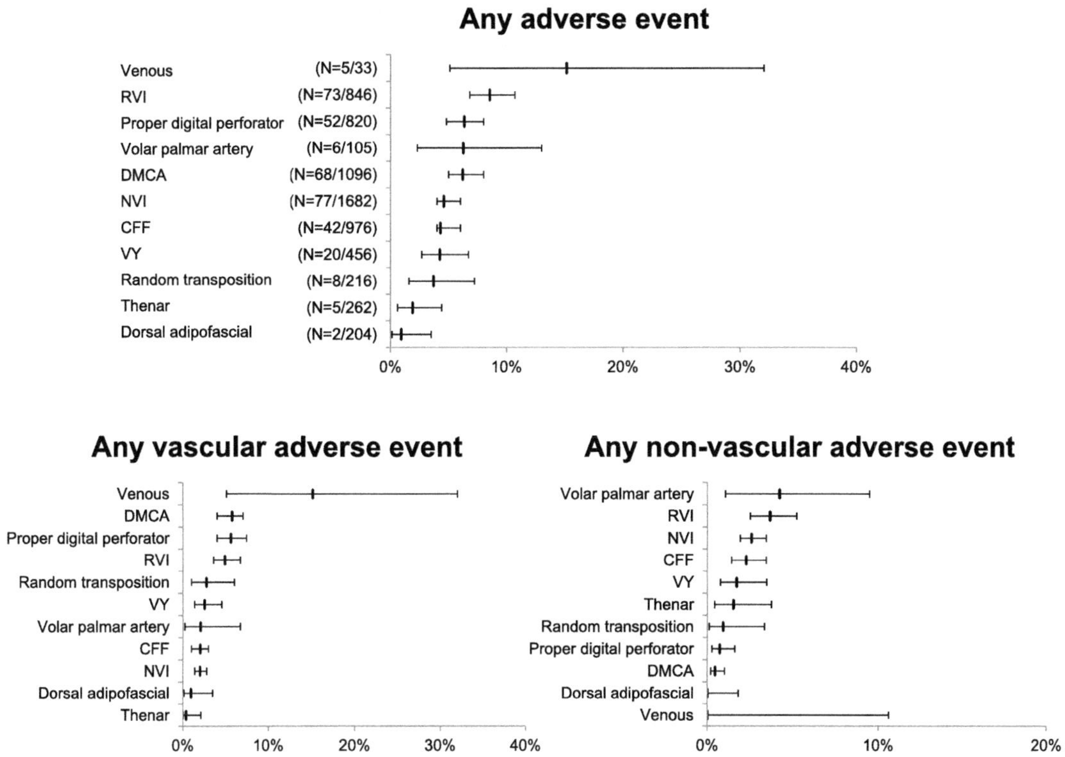

Fig. 2. Incidence proportions of adverse events for each flap type. Whiskers represent 95% CI.

Table 4
Nonvascular complications by flap type

Flap	Flaps, n	Donor Site	Scar Contracture	Pain Problem	Infection	Bulkiness	Inadequate Cover	Total
CFF	976	0.8	0.1	0.3	0.4	0.5	0.1	2.3
DMCA	1096	0.2	0	0	0.3	0	0	0.5
Dorsal adipofascial	204	0	0	0	0	0	0	0
NVI	1682	0.1	0.2	0.7	1.4	0	0.3	2.7
Digital perforator	820	0	0.1	0	0.1	0.5	0	0.7
Random transposition	216	0	0.9	0	0	0	0	0.9
RVI	846	0.5	1.2	0.7	0.7	0.5	0.1	3.7
Thenar	262	0.7	0.4	0.4	0	0	0	1.5
Venous	33	0	0	0	0	0	0	0
Volar palmar	105	0	3.8	0	0	0	0	3.8
VY-plasty	456	0	0	0.2	1.5	0	0	1.7

Data are expressed as percentages.

Abbreviations: CFF, cross finger flap; DMCA, dorsal metacarpal artery–based flap; NVI, neurovascular island flap; RVI, reverse vascular island flap.

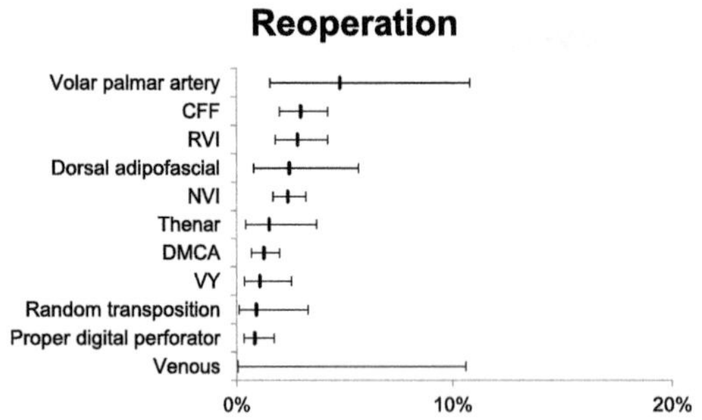

Fig. 3. Rate of reoperations for each flap type. Whiskers represent 95% CI.

DISCUSSION

Vascular Events

In the published reports, the average rate of adverse events in hand flap operations was 5.4% and vascular compromise was the most common reported adverse event comprising two-thirds of all complications. Vascular compromise occurred most commonly with perforator-based flaps or reverse flow flaps (digital artery perforator, DMCA, or RVI flap). The finding is plausible as the perfusion of these flaps is tenuous and venous return is easily compromised. In mild cases, this results in epidermolysis (not recorded in this review), but in more severe cases partial loss of flap may occur.

Dorsal adipofascial flaps and flaps with skin pedicle showed the lowest risk for vascular compromise. This is likely related to the short transposition distance and the robust vascular supply provided by the wide base in these flaps. Based on this meta-analysis, homodigital dorsal adipofascial flaps seem to be a reliable option for dorsal defects and they do not harm adjacent fingers.

Vascular insufficiency seldom (<1% of the flaps) caused complete loss of flap. It is likely that complete loss of flap is often primarily caused by arterial compromise. The tissue composition may also contribute to the rate of total failures. The dorsal adipofascial turnover flaps were reliable and this may be due to the absence of skin, resulting in lower metabolic rate and incidence of ischemic complications.

The incidence of complications varied from 1% to 10%, with most of the flaps and considering that trauma causing the defects also contributes to the adverse events, the reoperation rates were low. Overall, the incidences were low and we consider the observed differences mostly unimportant in clinical practice.

Non-Vascular Events

The non-vascular events dispersed among the flaps. Flaps raised from fingers (RVI and NVI flaps and CFF) may cause more pain-related complications compared with flaps raised from dorsum of the hand but their indications are also different. This finding may be associated with the recipient site. Flaps used for fingertip reconstruction exhibit hypersensitivity because the area is densely innervated. Furthermore, flaps that require incisions across the glabrous skin (NVI, RVI and volar transposition flaps) seemed to exhibit the highest rate of scar contractures.

Certainty of Evidence

Some of the variation may be explained by the sample size. Neurovascular island flaps (n = 1682 in 52 studies) comprised 25% of all flaps in our meta-analysis and 5 most common flap types (NVI, DMCA, CFF, RVI, and proper digital perforator flaps) comprised 80% of all flaps. The highest and lowest frequencies were reported in flaps with the lowest number (venous, volar palmar artery, and dorsal adipofascial flap), which comprise only 5% of all flaps. Small samples are statically more likely to exhibit extreme proportions. It is also possible that high incidence is associated with the small number of performed procedures (ie, learning curve). Furthermore, small sample size caused wide 95% CI for adverse events and reoperation rates indicating imprecision of the mean estimate.

Loss of flap is directly related to the reconstruction itself and will not occur in participants without flap surgery. Other complications can occur also due to trauma or after other type of tissue coverage. Thus, the reported incidences of non-vascular events should not be fully considered as flap-related complications but more as complications related to complex trauma and reconstructive surgery. Only rigorously conducted large RCTs would yield precise estimates.

In the studies included in this meta-analysis, adverse events were generally reported without any specific period for follow-up. We must assume that the duration of follow-up period varied significantly between studies and therefore it is impossible to estimate exact incidence rates (incidence during a specific time period). However, vascular adverse events usually occur within a the immediate follow-up period,[5] and were likely reported more comprehensively than the other adverse events presenting later and thus not be included in the studies.

All said, our estimates of vascular complications likely reflect the magnitude they are met in clinical practice. Flap necrosis cannot occur without flap procedure, and the cohorts consistently reported these events; fewer than 4% of all potentially eligible studies had to be excluded due to lack of reporting of vascular events, suggesting reasonable reporting of this outcome. Lack of considerable inconsistency in the estimates within flap types also imply reliable rates. However, we acknowledge the possibility of survivorship bias (cohorts including only survived flaps).

Implications for Practice

We did not formally compare the adverse event rates between the flap types, as we did not identify any RCTs and there was likely both clinical diversity and heterogeneous reporting in the studies. Trauma-related factors such as defect size and location likely affect the rates of most types of adverse events in this review. Because the incidence of adverse events was low in all flap types, one should primarily choose the flap based on considerations other than risk for adverse event (eg, defect size, location, need for skin sensation, and donor site morbidity).

However, when not guided by other considerations, one can always choose a flap with smaller risk of adverse events. An example would be a dorsal digital defect, which could be covered with a dorsal adipofascial turnover flap instead of DMCA-based flap, all other things being equal. Similarly, if VY-plasty, volar transposition flap, or NVI flap can cover a small volar defect, RVI flap would not be a preferred option due to higher vascular complication rate, and CFF due to higher rate of nonvascular complications, most notably donor site morbidity and bulkiness.

Volar scar contractures may be avoided by carefully planning the incisions and avoiding linear closures. Also, skin grafts are useful in donor site closure and probably can avoid tight scars in volar-lateral raised RVI flaps. Furthermore, when covering proximal pulp defects with advancement flaps, one should pay attention to digital nerve endings so that they are not left in the distal wound and develop painful neuromas of the tip. However, it is not clear if the neuropathic pain can be reliably avoided by any intervention.

Finally, the estimates from this study can be used to inform patients before surgery about the estimated rates of adverse events as well as need for reoperations.

Implications for Research

We could identify only one RCT and it did not report adverse events.[240] Also, the randomization was compromised as the groups were not comparable at the baseline. RCTs are hard to power adequately to detect differences in rare events. A large registry designed to systematically record adverse events would be a more feasible approach and yield more reliable estimates compared with pooling data from heterogeneous cohorts.

Future trials on local pedicled flap reconstruction should carefully define the complications a priori and report them systematically. Some complications, such as too bulky flaps or inadequate cover, may be better assessed with condition or area-specific patient-reported outcome measures (for example, Michigan Hand Questionnaire[241] or Cold Intolerance Symptom Severity questionnaire[242]). Flexion contractures can be assessed objectively by measuring range of motion, whereas disability may be best assessed with a patient-rated outcome measure instead of goniometer.[243] Loss of flap, reoperation, and infection are probably best assessed using binary outcome, although exact criteria for postoperative surgical site infection are notoriously difficult to define.

REFERENCES

1. Al-Qattan MM. The cross-digital dorsal adipofascial flap. Ann Plast Surg 2008;60(2):150–3.
2. Al-Qattan MM. Time of return back to work and complications following cross-finger flaps in industrial workers: comparison between immediate post operative mobilization versus immobilization until flap division. Int J Surg Case Rep 2018;42:70–4.
3. Gokrem S, Tuncali D, Terzioglu A, et al. The thin cross finger skin flap. J Hand Surg Eur Vol 2007; 32(4):417–20.
4. Johnson RK, Iverson RE. Cross-finger pedicle flaps in the hand. J Bone Joint Surg Am 1971;53(5): 913–9.
5. Karjalainen TV, Sebastin SJ, Chee KG, et al. Flap related complications requiring secondary surgery in a series of 851 local flaps used for fingertip reconstruction. J Hand Surg Asian Pac Vol 2019; 24(1):1–6.
6. Kleinert HE, McAlister CG, MacDonald CJ, et al. A critical evaluation of cross finger flaps. J Trauma 1974;14(9):756–63.
7. Lassner F, Becker M, Berger A, et al. Sensory reconstruction of the fingertip using the bilaterally innervated sensory cross-finger flap. Plast Reconstr Surg 2002;109(3):988–93.
8. Lee N-H, Pae W-S, Roh S-G, et al. Innervated cross-finger pulp flap for reconstruction of the fingertip. Arch Plast Surg 2012;39(6):637–42.
9. Lu J, Cui H, Zhang W, et al. Repair of degloving injury of fingertip with vascular pedicled cross

finger flap. Zhongguo Xiu Fu Chong Jian Wai Ke Za Zhi 2013;27(12):1480–3 [in Chinese].
10. Megerle K, Palm-Broking K, Germann G. The cross-finger flap. Oper Orthop Traumatol 2008; 20(2):97–102 [in German].
11. Mishra S, Manisundaram S. A reverse flow cross finger pedicle skin flap from hemidorsum of finger. J Plast Reconstr Aesthet Surg 2010;63(4):686–92.
12. Mutaf M, Sensoz O, Ustuner ET. A new design of the cross-finger flap: the C-ring flap. Br J Plast Surg 1993;46(2):97–104.
13. Al-Qattan M, Al-Turaiki T. Flexor tendon repair in zone 2 using a six-strand "figure of eight" suture. J Hand Surg Eur Vol 2009;34(3):322–8.
14. Paterson P, Titley OG, Nancarrow JD. Donor finger morbidity in cross-finger flaps. Injury 2000;31(4): 215–8.
15. Rabarin F, Saint Cast Y, Jeudy J, et al. Cross-finger flap for reconstruction of fingertip amputations: long-term results. Orthop Traumatol Surg Res 2016;102(4 Suppl):S225–8.
16. Sabapathy SR, Mohan D, Bharathi RR. "Jumping" cross finger flaps: a useful technique for salvaging parts in mutilating hand injuries. Br J Plast Surg 2000;53(6):488–90.
17. Saraf S, Tiwari V. Fingertip injuries. Indian J Orthop 2007;41(2):163.
18. Thomson HG, Sorokolit WT. The cross-finger flap in children: a follow-up study. Plast Reconstr Surg 1967;39(5):482–7.
19. Venkataswami R, Gnanasekaran TC. The staged Island flap: a new method of repair for thumb injuries. J Hand Surg Am 1990;15 B(4):425–8.
20. Vlastou C, Earle AS, Blanchard JM. A palmar cross-finger flap for coverage of thumb defects. J Hand Surg Am 1985;10(4):566–9.
21. Walker MA, Hurley CB, May JW Jr. Radial nerve cross-finger flap differential nerve contribution in thumb reconstruction. J Hand Surg Am 1986; 11(6):881–7.
22. Wang B, Zhang X, Jiang W, et al. Reconstruction of distally degloved fingers with a cross-finger flap and a composite-free flap from the dorsum of the second toe. J Hand Surg Am 2012;37(2): 303–9.e4.
23. Woon CY, Lee JY, Teoh LC. Resurfacing hemipulp losses of the thumb: the cross finger flap revisited: indications, technical refinements, outcomes, and long-term neurosensory recovery. Ann Plast Surg 2008;61(4):385–91.
24. Al-Qattan MM. De-epithelialized cross-finger flaps versus adipofascial turnover flaps for the reconstruction of small complex dorsal digital defects: a comparative analysis. J Hand Surg Am 2005; 30(3):549–57.
25. Shao X, Chen C, Zhang X, et al. Coverage of fingertip defect using a dorsal island pedicle flap including both dorsal digital nerves. J Hand Surg Am 1904;34(8):1474–81.
26. Atasoy E. The cross thumb to index finger pedicle. J Hand Surg Am 1980;5(6):572–4.
27. Bralliar F, Horner RL. Sensory cross-finger pedicle graft. J Bone Joint Surg Am 1969;51(7):1264–8.
28. Chen C, Tang P, Zhang L, et al. Treatment of fingertip degloving injury using the bilaterally innervated sensory cross-finger flap. Ann Plast Surg 2014;73(6):645–51.
29. Chong CW, Lin CH, Lin YT, et al. Refining the cross-finger flap: considerations of flap insetting, aesthetics and donor site morbidity. J Plast Reconstr Aesthet Surg 2018;71(4):566–72.
30. Dabernig J, Hart AM, Schwabegger AH, et al. Evaluation outcome of replanted digits using the DASH score: review of 38 patients. Int J Surg 2005;4(1): 30–6.
31. Erken HY, Akmaz I, Takka S, et al. Reconstruction of the transverse and dorsal-oblique amputations of the distal thumb with volar cross-finger flap using the index finger. J Hand Surg Eur Vol 2015; 40(4):392–400.
32. El Andaloussi Y, Fnini S, Labsaili A, et al. The Foucher's "kite-flap" (12 cases). Chir Main 2007; 26(1):31–4 [in French].
33. Benito JR, Ferreres A, Rodriguez-Baeza A, et al. Is the reversed fourth dorsal metacarpal flap reliable? J Hand Surg Am 2000;25 B(2):135–9.
34. Ege A, Tuncay I, Ercetin O. Foucher's first dorsal metacarpal artery flap for thumb reconstruction: evaluation of 21 cases. Isr Med Assoc J 2002; 4(6):421–3.
35. Ekerot L. The distally-based dorsal hand flap for resurfacing skin defects in Dupuytren's contracture. J Hand Surg Br 1995;20(1):111–4.
36. El-Khatib HA. Clinical experiences with the extended first dorsal metacarpal artery island flap for thumb reconstruction. J Hand Surg Am 1998; 23(4):647–52.
37. Foucher G, Braun JB. A new island flap transfer from the dorsum of the index to the thumb. Plast Reconstr Surg 1979;63(3):344–9.
38. Hussain A, Saleem A, Yasir M, et al. Comparison of first dorsal metacarpal artery flap done by consultants and residents and guidelines for improving outcome for beginners. Int J Res Med Sci 2016; 4(10):4310–3.
39. Karacalar A, Ozcan M. Second dorsal metacarpal artery neurovascular island flap: clinical applications. Eur J Plast Surg 1995;18(4):153–6.
40. Karacalar A, Ozcan M. A new approach to the reverse dorsal metacarpal artery flap. J Hand Surg Am 1997;22(2):307–10.
41. Karacalar A, Akin S, Ozcan M. The second dorsal metacarpal artery flap with double pivot points. Br J Plast Surg 1996;49(2):97–102.

42. Karamürsel S, Kayikçioğlu A, Aksoy HM, et al. Dorsal visor flap in fingertip reconstruction. Plast Reconstr Surg 2001;108(4):1014–8.
43. Karamürsel S, Celebioğlu S. Reverse-flow first dorsal metacarpal artery flap for index fingertip reconstruction. Ann Plast Surg 2005;54(6):600–3.
44. Chang SC, Chen SL, Chen TM, et al. Sensate first dorsal metacarpal artery flap for resurfacing extensive pulp defects of the thumb. Ann Plast Surg 2004;53(5):449–54.
45. Koch H, Bruckmann L, Hubmer M, et al. Extended reverse dorsal metacarpal artery flap: clinical experience and donor site morbidity. Br J Plast Surg 2006;60(4):349–55.
46. Lai-Jin L, Xu G. The reverse dorsal metacarpal flap: experience with 153 cases. Ann Plast Surg 2006; 56(6):614–7.
47. Legaillard P, Grangier Y, Casoli V, et al. Boomerang flap. A real one-stage cross-finger pedicle flap. Ann Chir Plast Esthet 1996;41(3):251–8 [in French].
48. Lu LJ, Gong X, Liu ZG, et al. Retrospective study of reverse dorsal metacarpal flap and compound flap: a review of 122 cases. Chin J Traumatol 2006;9(1):21–4.
49. Ramy M. The innervated first dorsal metacarpal artery island flap for reconstruction of post-traumatic thumb defect. Eur J Plast Surg 2012;35:881–6.
50. Shehata Ibrahim Ahmed M, Salah Ibrahim E, Ibrahim Eltayeb H. Evaluation of versatility of use of island first dorsal metacarpal artery flap in reconstruction of dorsal hand defects. Asian J Surg 2019;42(1):197–202.
51. Maruyama Y. The reverse dorsal metacarpal flap. Br J Plast Surg 1989;43(1):24–7.
52. Molski M. First dorsal metacarpal flap in compound multi tissues thumb reconstruction. Chir Narzadow Ruchu Ortop Pol 2003;68(2):115–9 [in Polish].
53. Muyldermans T, Hierner R. First dorsal metacarpal artery flap for thumb reconstruction: a retrospective clinical study. Strategies Trauma Limb Reconstr 2009;4(1):27–33.
54. Pagliei A, Rocchi L, Tulli A. The dorsal flap of the first web. J Hand Surg Am 2003;28 B(2):121–4.
55. Chen SL, Chou TD, Chen SG, et al. The boomerang flap in managing injuries of the dorsum of the distal phalanx. Plast Reconstr Surg 2000;106(4):834–9.
56. Carolina Posso Z, David Delgado A, Jeison Aguilar H, et al. Second dorsal metacarpal artery perforator flap: anatomical study and clinical experience. Rev Iberoam Cir La Mano 2018;46(1):3–11 [in Spanish].
57. Qian J, Rui Y, Zhang Q, et al. Effectiveness of dorsal metacarpal island flap for treating scar contracture of finger web. Zhongguo Xiu Fu Chong Jian Wai Ke Za Zhi 2011;25(11):1347–9 [in Chinese].
58. Quaba AA, Davison PM. The distally-based dorsal hand flap. Br J Plast Surg 1989;43(1):28–39.
59. Ratcliffe RJ, Regan PJ, Scerri GV. First dorsal metacarpal artery flap cover for extensive pulp defects in the normal length thumb. Br J Plast Surg 1992; 45(7):544–6.
60. Saalabian A, Rab M, van Schoonhoven J, et al. Foucher's first dorsal metacarpal artery island flap. Oper Orthop Traumatol 2009;21(6):614–9 [in German].
61. Satish C, Nema S. First dorsal metacarpal artery islanded flap: a useful flap for reconstruction of thumb pulp defects. Indian J Plast Surg 2009; 42(1):32.
62. Schoofs M, Chambon E, Leps P, et al. The reverse dorsal metacarpal flap from the first web. Eur J Plast Surg 1993;16(1):26–9.
63. Sebastin S, Mendoza R, Chong A, et al. Application of the dorsal metacarpal artery perforator flap for resurfacing soft-tissue defects proximal to the fingertip. Plast Reconstr Surg 2011;128(3): 166e–78e.
64. Shen H, Shen Z, Wang Y, et al. Extended reverse dorsal metacarpal artery flap for coverage of finger defects distal to the proximal interphalangeal joint. Ann Plast Surg 2014;72(5):529–36.
65. Jing H, Liu XY, Ge BF, et al. The second dorsal metacarpal flap with vascular pedicle composed of the second dorsal metacarpal artery and the dorsal carpal branch of radial artery. Plast Reconstr Surg 1993;92(3):501–6.
66. Chen C, Zhang X, Shao X, et al. Treatment of thumb tip degloving injury using the modified first dorsal metacarpal artery flap. J Hand Surg Am 2010; 35(10):1663–70.
67. Small JO, Brennen MD. The second dorsal metacarpal artery neurovascular island flap. Br J Plast Surg 1990;43(1):17–23.
68. Small JO, Brennen MD. The first dorsal metacarpal artery neurovascular island flap. J Hand Surg Br 1988;13(2):136–45.
69. Song JL. The third dorsal metacarpal artery neuromuscular island flap. Zhonghua Zheng Xing Shao Shang Wai Ke Za Zhi 1993;9(3):204–5, 238-9. [in Chinese].
70. Vuppalapati G, Oberlin C, Balakrishnan G. "Distally based dorsal hand flaps": clinical experience, cadaveric studies and an update. Br J Plast Surg 2004;57(7):653–67.
71. Wang H, Chen C, Li J, et al. Modified first dorsal metacarpal artery island flap for sensory reconstruction of thumb pulp defects. J Hand Surg Eur Vol 2016;41(2):177–84.
72. Yang JY. The first dorsal metacarpal flap in first web space and thumb reconstruction. Ann Plast Surg 1991;27(3):258–64.
73. Yousif NJ, Ye Z, Sanger JR, et al. The versatile metacarpal and reverse metacarpal artery flaps in hand surgery. Ann Plast Surg 1992;29(6):523–31.

74. Zhang X, He Y, Shao X, et al. Second dorsal metacarpal artery flap from the dorsum of the middle finger for coverage of volar thumb defect. J Hand Surg Am 2009;34(8):1467–73.
75. Zhang X, Shao X, Ren C, et al. Reconstruction of thumb pulp defects using a modified kite flap. J Hand Surg Am 2011;36(10):1597–603.
76. Zhang X, Yang L, Shao X, et al. Use of a bilobed second dorsal metacarpal artery-based island flap for thumb replantation. J Hand Surg Am 2011;36(6):998–1006.
77. Chen C, Zhang X, Shao X, et al. Treatment of a combination of volar soft tissue and proper digital nerve defects using the dorsal digital nerve island flap. J Hand Surg Am 2010;35(10):1655–62.e3.
78. Zhang W, Zhao G, Gao S, et al. Anatomy study and clinical application of island flap based on second dorsal metacarpal artery. Zhonghua Zheng Xing Wai Ke Za Zhi 2016;32(2):118–21 [in Chinese].
79. Zhang W, Zhang Z, Gao S, et al. Repair of finger tissue defect with modified island flap based on reversed dorsal metacarpal artery. Zhongguo Xiu Fu Chong Jian Wai Ke Za Zhi 2010;24(6):718–21 [in Chinese].
80. Zhang W, Jiao C, Liu Y. Repair of finger soft tissue defect with island flap based on vascular chain of cutaneous branch of dorsal metacarpal artery. Zhongguo Xiu Fu Chong Jian Wai Ke Za Zhi 2013;27(4):440–2 [in Chinese].
81. Zhu H, Cao Y, Wan L, et al. Repair of deep wound on thumb using island flap from dorsoulnar side of thumb. Zhonghua Shao Shang Za Zhi 2014;30(5): 405–7 [in Chinese].
82. Zhu H, Zhang X, Yan M, et al. Treatment of complex soft-tissue defects at the metacarpophalangeal joint of the thumb using the bilobed second dorsal metacarpal artery-based island flap. Plast Reconstr Surg 2013;131(5):1091–7.
83. Chen C, Tang P, Zhang X. The dorsal homodigital island flap based on the dorsal branch of the digital artery: a review of 166 cases. Plast Reconstr Surg 2014;133(4):519e–29e.
84. Couceiro J, Sanmartin M. The Holevich flap revisited: a comparison with the Foucher flap, case series. Hand Surg 2014;19(3):469–74.
85. Duman H, Uygur F, Evinc R. The use of reverse-flow dorsal metacarpal artery flaps after postburn metacarpophalangeal joint flexion contracture release. Cent Eur J Med 2010;5(2):159–64.
86. Earley M. The second dorsal metacarpal artery neurovascular island flap. J Hand Surg Br 1989; 14(4):434–40.
87. Al-Qattan MM. The adipofascial turnover flap for coverage of the exposed distal interphalangeal joint of the fingers and interphalangeal joint of the thumb. J Hand Surg Am 2001;26(6):1116–9.
88. Al-Qattan MM. The use of adipofascial turnover flaps for coverage of complex dorsal ring finger defects caused by electric burns. Burns 2005;31(5): 643–6.
89. Al-Qattan MM. Technical modifications and extended applications of the distally based adipofascial flap for dorsal digital defects. Ann Plast Surg 2004;52(2):168–73.
90. Braga-Silva J, Kuyven CR, Albertoni W, et al. The adipofascial turn-over flap for coverage of the dorsum of the finger: a modified surgical technique. J Hand Surg Am 2004;29(6):1038–43.
91. Braga Silva J, Ramos RM, Piccinini PS. De-epithelialized dorsal digital turnover flap for coverage of volar digital lesions: a modified technique. Eur J Plast Surg 2017;40(5):479–82.
92. Camporro D, Vidal D, Robla D. Extended applications of distally based axial adipofascial flaps for hand and digits defects. J Plast Reconstr Aesthet Surg 2010;63(12):2117–22.
93. Delia G, Campolo MF, Risitano G, et al. Homodigital dorsal adipofascial reverse flap: clinical applications. Plast Reconstr Surg 2011;127(6):162e–3e.
94. Karamese M, Akatekin A, Abac M, et al. Fingertip reconstruction with reverse adipofascial homodigital flap. Ann Plast Surg 2015;75(2):158–62.
95. Lai CS, Lin SD, Yang CC, et al. The adipofascial turn-over flap for complicated dorsal skin defects of the hand and finger. Br J Plast Surg 1991; 44(3):165–9.
96. Laoulakos DH, Tsetsonis CH, Michail AA, et al. The dorsal reverse adipofascial flap for fingertip reconstruction. Plast Reconstr Surg 2003;112(1): 121–8.
97. Unlü RE, Mengi AS, Koçer U, et al. Dorsal adipofascial turn-over flap for fingertip amputations. J Hand Surg Br 1999;24(5):525–30.
98. Elliot D, Wilson Y. V-Y advancement of the entire volar soft tissue of the thumb in distal reconstruction. J Hand Surg Br 1993;18(3):399–402.
99. Evans DM, Martin DL. Step-advancement island flap for fingertip reconstruction. Br J Plast Surg 1988;41(2):105–11.
100. Foucher G, Delaere O, Citron N, et al. Long-term outcome of neurovascular palmar advancement flaps for distal thumb injuries. Br J Plast Surg 1999;52(1):64–8.
101. Foucher G, Smith D, Pempinello C, et al. Homodigital neurovascular island flaps for digital pulp loss. J Hand Surg Br 1989;14(2):204–8.
102. Gassmann N, Segmueller G. The neurovascular palmar advancement flap (MOBERG). Analysis of unsatisfactory results. Handchirurgie 1976;8(2): 77–80 [in German].
103. Gaul JS Jr. A palmar-hinged flap for reconstruction of traumatic thumb defects. J Hand Surg Am 1987; 12(3):415–21.

104. Hammouda AA, El-Khatib HA, Al-Hetmi T. Extended step-advancement flap for avulsed amputated fingertip–a new technique to preserve finger length: case series. J Hand Surg Am 2011; 36(1):129–34.
105. Henderson HP, Reid DAC. Long term follow up of neurovascular island flaps. Hand 1980;12(2): 113–22.
106. Hou CL. The use of a neurovascular island flap at the radial side of the index finger to repair a wound of the thumb tip. Zhonghua Zheng Xing Shao Shang Wai Ke Za Zhi 1986;2(3):197–8, 235. [in Chinese].
107. Iwasawa M, Kawamura T, Nagai F. Dorsally extended digital island flap for repairing soft tissue injury of the fingertip. J Plast Reconstr Aesthet Surg 2011;64(10):1300–5.
108. Adani R, Squarzina PB, Castagnetti C, et al. A comparative study of the heterodigital neurovascular island flap in thumb reconstruction, with and without nerve reconnection. J Hand Surg Am 1994;19 B(5):552–9.
109. Joshi BB. A local dorsolateral island flap for restoration of sensation after avulsion injury of fingertip pulp. Plast Reconstr Surg 1974;54(2):175–82.
110. Kapandji T, Bleton R, Alnot JY, et al. Digital flap autografts for pulp coverage in distal amputations of the fingers. 68 flaps. Ann Chir Main Memb Super 1991;10(5):406–16 [in French].
111. Kayalar M. The outcome of direct-flow neurovascular island flaps in pulp defects. Acta Orthop Traumatol Turc 2011;45(3):175–84.
112. Kumta SM, Yip KMH, Pannozzo A, et al. Resurfacing of thumb-pulp loss with a heterodigital neurovascular island flap using a nerve disconnection/reconnection technique. J Reconstr Microsurg 1997;13(2):117–23.
113. Lanzetta M, Mastropasqua B, Chollet A, et al. Versatility of the homodigital triangular neurovascular island flap in fingertip reconstruction. J Hand Surg Br 1995;20(6):824–9.
114. Lee YH, Baek GH, Gong HS, et al. Innervated lateral middle phalangeal finger flap for a large pulp defect by bilateral neurorrhaphy. Plast Reconstr Surg 2006;118(5):1185–93 [discussion: 1194].
115. Lim GJ, Yam AK, Lee JY, et al. The spiral flap for fingertip resurfacing: short-term and long-term results. J Hand Surg Am 2008;33(3):340–7.
116. Liu H, Regmi S, He Y, et al. Thumb tip defect reconstruction using neurovascular island pedicle flap obtained from long finger. Aesthetic Plast Surg 2016;40(5):755–60.
117. Loréa P, Chahidi N, Marchesi S, et al. Reconstruction of fingertip defects with the neurovascular tranquilli-leali flap. J Hand Surg Br 2006;31(3): 280–4.
118. Macht SD, Watson HK. The Moberg volar advancement flap for digital reconstruction. J Hand Surg Am 1980;5(4):372–6.
119. Adani R, Busa R, Castagnetti C, et al. Homodigital neurovascular island flaps with "direct flow" vascularization. Ann Plast Surg 1997;38(1):36–40.
120. Massart P, Saucier T, Bèzes H. Restoration of the pulp with a homodigital neurovascular flap. Ann Chir Main 1985;4(3):219–25.
121. Mouchet A, Gilbert A. Covering distal amputations of the finger using homodigital neurovascular island flaps. Ann Chir Main 1982;1(2):180–2 [in French].
122. Murray JF, Ord JV, Gavelin GE. The neurovascular island pedicle flap. An assessment of late results in sixteen cases. J Bone Joint Surg Am 1967;49(7): 1285–97.
123. Nakanishi A, Omokawa S, Iida A, et al. Predictors of proximal interphalangeal joint flexion contracture after homodigital island flap. J Hand Surg Am 2015;40(11):2155–9.
124. Noack N, Hartmann B, Germann G, et al. Fillet flaps as a possibility for defect reconstruction of the hand: reconstruction without additional donor site morbidity. Unfallchirurg 2005;108(4):293–8 [in German].
125. Oka Y. Sensory function of the neurovascular island flap in thumb reconstruction: comparison of original and modified procedures. J Hand Surg Am 2000;25(4):637–43.
126. Holevich J, Paneva-Holevich E. Bipedicled island flap. Acta Chir Plast 1971;13(2):106–16.
127. Pho RW. Local composite neurovascular island flap for skin cover in pulp loss of the thumb. J Hand Surg Am 1978;4(1):11–5.
128. Qian L, Zhang Q, Rui Y, et al. Repair of finger pulp defect with transverse digital palmar island flap. Zhongguo Xiu Fu Chong Jian Wai Ke Za Zhi 2009;23(10):1164–6 [in Chinese].
129. Schuind F, Van Genechten F, Denuit P. Homodigital neurovascular island flaps in hand surgery. A study of sixty cases. Ann Chir Main 1985;4(4):306–15 [in French].
130. Bakhach J, Guimberteau J, Panconi B. The gigogne flap: an original technique for an optimal pulp reconstruction. J Hand Surg Eur Vol 2009; 34(2):227–34.
131. Segmüller G. Modification of Kutler-Lappens: Neurovaskuläre Stielung. Handchir. Mikrochir. Plast Chir 1976;8:75–6.
132. Smith KL, Elliot D. The extended Segmüller flap. Plast Reconstr Surg 2000;105(4):1334–46.
133. Snow JW. The use of a volar flap for repair of fingertip amputations: a preliminary report. Comment. Plast Reconstr Surg 1973;52(3):299.

134. Stice RC, Wood MB. Neurovascular island skin flaps in the hand: functional and sensibility evaluations. Microsurgery 1987;8(3):162–7.
135. Teoh L-C, Tay SC, Yong FC, et al. Heterodigital arterialized flaps for large finger wounds: results and indications. Plast Reconstr Surg 2003; 111(6):1905–13.
136. Toros T, Gurbuz Y, Kelesoglu B, et al. Reconstruction of extensive pulp defects of the thumb with a radial-based pedicled flap from the index finger. J Hand Surg Eur Vol 2018;43(10):1036–43.
137. Usami S, Kawahara S, Yamaguchi Y, et al. Homodigital artery flap reconstruction for fingertip amputation: a comparative study of the oblique triangular neurovascular advancement flap and the reverse digital artery island flap. J Hand Surg Eur Vol 2015;40(3):291–7.
138. Varitimidis SE, Dailiana ZH, Zibis AH, et al. Restoration of function and sensitivity utilizing a homodigital neurovascular island flap after amputation injuries of the fingertip. J Hand Surg Br 2005; 30(4):338–42.
139. Venkataswami R, Subramanian N. Oblique triangular flap: a new method of repair for oblique amputations of the fingertip and thumb. Plast Reconstr Surg 1980;66(2):296–300.
140. Xarchas KC, Tilkeridis KE, Pelekas SI, et al. Littler's flap revisited: an anatomic study, literature review, and clinical experience in the reconstruction of large thumb-pulp defects. Med Sci Monit 2008; 14(11):CR568–73.
141. Baumeister S, Menke H, Wittemann M, et al. Functional outcome after the Moberg advancement flap in the thumb. J Hand Surg Am 2002;27(1):105–14.
142. Zhang Z, Yan BS, Wu XM, et al. Repair of finger pulp defect with the homodigital spiral neurovascular island flap. Zhongguo Gu Shang 2011;24(5): 422–4 [in Chinese].
143. Ozaksar K, Toros T, Sügün TS, et al. Reconstruction of finger pulp defects using homodigital dorsal middle phalangeal neurovascular advancement flap. J Hand Surg Eur Vol 2010;35(2):125–9.
144. Boe S. The neurovascular island pedicle flap. Acta Orthop Scand 1979;50(1):67–71.
145. Borman H, Maral T, Tancer M. Fingertip reconstruction using two variations of direct-flow homodigital neurovascular island flaps. Ann Plast Surg 2000; 45(1):24–30.
146. Chang S, Jin W, Wei Z, et al. Repair of skin and soft tissue defects at distal end of finger with serrated flap with digital proper artery and nerve pedicle combined with bilaterally pedicled V-Y advancement flap of the injured finger. Zhonghua Shao Shang Za Zhi 2016;32(4):204–7 [in Chinese].
147. Chen C, Zhang W, Tang P. Direct and reversed dorsal digito-metacarpal flaps: a review of 24 cases. Injury 2014;45(4):805–12.
148. Del Bene M. Reverse dorsal digital island flap. Plast Reconstr Surg 1994;93(3):552–7.
149. Hirase Y, Kojima T, Matsuura S. A versatile one-stage neurovascular flap for fingertip reconstruction: the dorsal middle phalangeal finger flap. Plast Reconstr Surg 1992;90(6):1009–15.
150. Keramidas E, Rodopoulou S, Metaxotos N, et al. Reverse dorsal digital and intercommissural flaps used for digital reconstruction. Br J Plast Surg 2004;57(1):61–5.
151. Kim KS, Yoo SI, Kim DY, et al. Fingertip reconstruction using a volar flap based on the transverse palmar branch of the digital artery. Ann Plast Surg 2001;47(3):263–8.
152. Koshima I, Urushibara K, Fukuda N, et al. Digital artery perforator flaps for fingertip reconstructions. Plast Reconstr Surg 2006;118(7):1579–84.
153. Mitsunaga N, Mihara M, Koshima I, et al. Digital artery perforator (DAP) flaps: modifications for fingertip and finger stump reconstruction. J Plast Reconstr Aesthet Surg 2010;63(8):1312–7.
154. Moschella F, Cordova A. Reverse homodigital dorsal radial flap of the thumb. Plast Reconstr Surg 2006;117(3):920–6.
155. Ozcanli H, Coskunfirat OK, Bektas G, et al. Innervated digital artery perforator flap. J Hand Surg Am 2013;38(2):350–6.
156. Ozcanli H, Cavit A. Innervated digital artery perforator flap: a versatile technique for fingertip reconstruction. J Hand Surg Am 2015;40(12):2352–7.
157. Pelissier P, Gardet H, Sawaya E, et al. Anatomical study of the palmar intermetacarpal perforator flap. J Hand Surg Eur Vol 2009;34(2):224–6.
158. Pelissier P, Casoli V, Bakhach J, et al. Reverse dorsal digital and metacarpal flaps: a review of 27 cases. Plast Reconstr Surg 1999;103(1):159–65.
159. Wei P, Chen W, Mei J, et al. Repair of fingertip defect using an anterograde pedicle flap based on the dorsal perforator. Plast Reconstr Surg Glob Open 2016;4(6):e730.
160. Shen XF, Xue MY, Mi JY, et al. Innervated digital artery perforator propeller flap for reconstruction of lateral oblique fingertip defects. J Hand Surg Am 2015;40(7):1382–8.
161. Shibu MM, Tarabe MA, Graham K, et al. Fingertip reconstruction with a dorsal island homodigital flap. Br J Plast Surg 1997;50(2):121–4.
162. Sun YC, Chen QZ, Chen J, et al. Reverse dorsoradial flaps for thumb coverage show increased sensory recovery with smaller flap sizes. J Reconstr Microsurg 2015;31(6):426–33.
163. Teran P, Carnero S, Miranda R, et al. Refinements in dorsoulnar flap of the thumb: 15 cases. J Hand Surg Am 2010;35(8):1356–9.

164. Vogelin E, Buchler U. Retrograde (neuro) vascular island flaps from the dorsum of the finger. Tech Hand Up Extrem Surg 2001;5(2):78–84.
165. Xianyu M, Lei C, Laijin L, et al. Reconstruction of finger-pulp defect with a homodigital laterodorsal fasciocutaneous flap distally based on the dorsal branches of the proper palmar digital artery. Injury 2009;40(12):1346–50.
166. Zhang X, Shao X, Zhu M, et al. Repair of a palmar soft tissue defect of the proximal interphalangeal joint with a transposition flap from the dorsum of the proximal phalanx. J Hand Surg Eur Vol 2013; 38(4):378–85.
167. Basat SO, Ugurlu AM, Aydin A, et al. Digital artery perforator flaps: an easy and reliable choice for fingertip amputation reconstruction. Acta Orthop Traumatol Turc 2013;47(4):250–4.
168. Zhou X, Xu Y, Rui Y, et al. Clinical application of island flap pedicled with dorsal cutaneous branches of thumb radial digital artery. Zhongguo Xiu Fu Chong Jian Wai Ke Za Zhi 2011;25(9):1036–9 [in Chinese].
169. Zhou X, Xu Y, Rui Y, et al. Application of distal palm perforator mini-flap in repair of scar contracture of digital web-spaces. Zhongguo Xiu Fu Chong Jian Wai Ke Za Zhi 2011;25(2):206–8 [in Chinese].
170. Bertelli JA, Pagliei A. Direct and reversed flow proximal phalangeal island flaps. J Hand Surg Am 1994;19(4):671–80.
171. Brunelli F, Brunelli G, Vigasio A. Dorso-ulnar thumb flap. Anatomical study and clinical application. Report of twenty-two cases. Ann Chir Plast Esthet 1996;41(3):259–68 [in French].
172. Brunelli F, Vigasio A, Valenti P, et al. Arterial anatomy and clinical application of the dorsoulnar flap of the thumb. J Hand Surg Am 1999;24(4): 803–11.
173. Chen C, Tang P, Zhang X. A comparison of the dorsal digital island flap with the dorsal branch of the digital nerve versus the dorsal digital nerve for fingertip and finger pulp reconstruction. Plast Reconstr Surg 2014;133(2):165e–73e.
174. Chen C, Tang P, Zhang L, et al. Repair of multiple finger defects using the dorsal homodigital island flaps. Injury 2013;44(11):1582–8.
175. Chen C, Tang P, Zhao G. Direct and reversed dorsal digital island flaps: a review of 65 cases. Injury 2014;45(12):2013–7.
176. Acikel C, Peker F, Yuksel F, et al. Bilateral side finger transposition flaps in the treatment of chronic postburn flexion contractures of the fingers. Ann Plast Surg 2002;49(4):344–9.
177. Foucher G, Dallaserra M, Tilquin B, et al. The Hueston flap in reconstruction of fingertip skin loss: results in a series of 41 patients. J Hand Surg Am 1994;19(3):508–15.
178. Souquet R. The asymmetric arterial advancement flap in distal pulp loss (modified Hueston's flap. Ann Chir Main 1985;4(3):233–8.
179. Sungur N, Kankaya Y, Yildiz K, et al. Bilateral V–Y rotation advancement flap for fingertip amputations. Hand 2012;7(1):79–85.
180. Tuncali D, Barutcu AY, Gokrem S, et al. The hatchet flap for reconstruction of fingertip amputations. Plast Reconstr Surg 2006;117(6):1933–9.
181. Xiu Z, Song Y. The dorsal fasciocutaneous island flap of the finger for the repair of volar skin defects of the same finger. Zhonghua Zheng Xing Wai Ke Za Zhi 2002;18(3):151–2 [in Chinese].
182. Yii NW, Elliot D. Bipedicle strap flaps in reconstruction of longitudinal dorsal skin defects of the digits. Plast Reconstr Surg 1999;103(4):1205–11.
183. Ozturk MB, Barutca SA, Aksan T, et al. Pulp rotation flap for lateral oblique fingertip defects. Ann Plast Surg 2016;77(5):529–34.
184. Germann G, Rütschle S, Kania N, et al. The reverse pedicle heterodigital cross-finger island flap. J Hand Surg Br 1997;22(1):25–9.
185. Hamdi MF, Sbai MA. The reversed homodigital island flap: 28 cases. Chir Main 2010;29(4):249–54 [in French].
186. Han SK, Lee BI, Kim WK. The reverse digital artery island flap: clinical experience in 120 fingers. Plast Reconstr Surg 1998;101(4):1006–11 [discussion: 1012–3].
187. Hu HT, Chen WH, Liu WC, et al. Fingertip reconstruction using a volar flap based on the transverse palmar branch of the digital artery. Zhonghua Zheng Xing Wai Ke Za Zhi 2005;21(5):353–5 [in Chinese].
188. Huang Y-C, Liu Y, Chen T-H. Use of homodigital reverse island flaps for distal digital reconstruction. J Trauma 2010;68(2):429–33.
189. Kaleli T, Ersozlu S, Ozturk C. Double reverse-flow island flaps for two adjacent finger tissue defect. Arch Orthop Trauma Surg 2004;124(3):157–60.
190. Kim J, Lee YH, Kim MB, et al. Innervated reverse digital artery island flap through bilateral neurorrhaphy using direct small branches of the proper digital nerve. Plast Reconstr Surg 2015;135(6): 1643–50.
191. Kojima T, Tsuchida Y, Hirase Y, et al. Reverse vascular pedicle digital island flap. Br J Plast Surg 1990;43(3):290–5.
192. Kayalar M, Bal E, Toros T, et al. The results of reverse-flow island flaps in pulp reconstruction. Acta Orthop Traumatol Turc 2011;45(5):304–11.
193. Lai CS, Lin SD, Yang CC. The reverse digital artery flap for fingertip reconstruction. Ann Plast Surg 1989;22(6):495–500.
194. Acar MA, Güzel Y, Güleç A, et al. Reconstruction of multiple fingertip injuries with reverse flow homodigital flap. Injury 2014;45(10):1569–73.

195. Lai CS, Lin SD, Chou CK, et al. A versatile method for reconstruction of finger defects: reverse digital artery flap. Br J Plast Surg 1992;45(6):443–53.
196. Lin BJ, Shih JT, Lee HM. Clinical experience using a reverse homodigital island flap in nearby fingertip reconstruction. J Med Sci 2007;27(3):109–12.
197. Liu G, Xi Z, Wang C, et al. Reverse island flap of digital artery parallel for repairing degloved injuries of fingertip. Zhongguo Xiu Fu Chong Jian Wai Ke Za Zhi 2011;25(9):1030–2 [in Chinese].
198. Matsuzaki H, Kouda H, Yamashita H. Preventing postoperative congestion in reverse pedicle digital island flaps when reconstructing composite tissue defects in the fingertip: a patient series. Hand Surg 2012;17(1):77–82.
199. Momeni A, Zajonc H, Kalash Z, et al. Reconstruction of distal phalangeal injuries with the reverse homodigital island flap. Injury 2008;39(12): 1460–3.
200. Niranjan NS, Armstrong JR. A homodigital reverse pedicle island flap in soft tissue reconstruction of the finger and the thumb. J Hand Surg Br 1994; 19(2):135–41.
201. Sapp JW, Allen RJ, Dupin C. A reversed digital artery island flap for the treatment of fingertip injuries. J Hand Surg Am 1993;18(3):528–34.
202. Takeishi M, Shinoda A, Sugiyama A, et al. Innervated reverse dorsal digital island flap for fingertip reconstruction. J Hand Surg Am 2006;31(7): 1094–9.
203. Tan O. Reverse dorsolateral proximal phalangeal island flap: a new versatile technique for coverage of finger defects. J Plast Reconstr Aesthet Surg 2010;63(1):146–52.
204. Xie HJ, Liu YF, Li HC, et al. Reverse-flow island flap transplantation of radialis dorsal digital artery for index finger defect. J Clin Rehabil Tissue Eng Res 2007;11(29):5668–71 [in Chinese].
205. Adani R, Marcuzzi A, Busa R, et al. Homodigital island flap with reverse vascular pedicle. A series of 15 cases and a review of the literature. Ann Chir Main Memb Super 1995;14(3):169–81 [in French].
206. Yazar M. Sensory recovery of the reverse homodigital island flap in fingertip reconstruction: a review of 66 cases. Acta Orthop Traumatol Turc 2010; 44(5):345–51.
207. Yildirim S, Avci G, Akan M, et al. Complications of the reverse homodigital island flap in fingertip reconstruction. Ann Plast Surg 2002;48(6): 586–92.
208. Xiao Z, Mingyu X, Yajun X, et al. Reconstruction of soft tissue defects at finger tip with relay flaps pedicled by perforator from digital artery. Zhonghua Zheng Xing Wai Ke Za Zhi 2015;31(6):422–5 [in Chinese].
209. Adani R, Busa R, Pancaldi G, et al. Reverse neurovascular homodigital island flap. Ann Plast Surg 1995;35(1):77–82.
210. Adani R, Marcoccio I, Tarallo L, et al. The reverse heterodigital neurovascular island flap for digital pulp reconstruction. Tech Hand Up Extrem Surg 2005;9(2):91–5.
211. Alagoz MS, Uysal CA, Kerem M, et al. Reverse homodigital artery flap coverage for bone and nailbed grafts in fingertip amputations. Ann Plast Surg 2006;56(3):279–83.
212. Chen QZ, Sun YC, Chen J, et al. Comparative study of functional and aesthetically outcomes of reverse digital artery and reverse dorsal homodigital island flaps for fingertip repair. J Hand Surg Eur Vol 2015;40(9):935–43.
213. Deng C, Wei Z, Sun G, et al. Repair of skin and soft tissue defects at distal end of finger and donor site with relaying reversed perforator flaps. Zhonghua Shao Shang Za Zhi 2015;31(2):107–11 [in Chinese].
214. Du Y, Feng X, Xu G. Clinical application of the reversed digital arterial island flap with digital vein and digital dorsal nerve anastomosis. Zhonghua Zheng Xing Wai Ke Za Zhi 2001;17(5):267–8 [in Chinese].
215. Ameziane L, Filali-Ansary N, El Manouar M. The thenar flap. Lyon Chir 1997;93(5):312–4 [in French].
216. Garcia Ariz M, Otero Lopez A, Otero Lopez ER, et al. Fingertip reconstruction with the "shark mouth" incision thenar flap: analysis of outcomes in pediatric patients. Bol Asoc Med P R 2014; 106(4):11–6.
217. Barbato BD, Guelmi K, Romano SJ, et al. Thenar flap rehabilitated: a review of 20 cases. Ann Plast Surg 1996;37(2):135–9.
218. Barr JS, Chu MW, Thanik V, et al. Pediatric thenar flaps: A modified design, case series and review of the literature. J Pediatr Surg 2014;49(9): 1433–8.
219. Dellon AL. The proximal inset thenar flap for fingertip reconstruction. Plast Reconstr Surg 1983;72(5):703–4.
220. Fitoussi F, Ghorbani A, Jehanno P, et al. Thenar flap for severe finger tip injuries in children. J Hand Surg Am 2004;29 B(2):108–12.
221. Melone CP, Beasley RW, Carstens JH. The thenar flap–an analysis of its use in 150 cases. J Hand Surg Am 1982;7(3):291–7.
222. Okazaki M, Hasegawa H, Kano M, et al. A different method of fingertip reconstruction with the thenar flap. Plast Reconstr Surg 2005; 115(3):885–8.
223. Smith JR, Bom AF. An evaluation of finger-tip reconstruction by cross-finger and palmar pedicle flap. Plast Reconstr Surg 1965;35:409–18.

224. Rinker B. Fingertip reconstruction with the laterally based thenar flap: indications and long-term functional results. Hand (N Y) 2006;1(1):2–8.
225. Gu JH, Han SK, Jeong SH, et al. Hand coverage using venous island flaps. J Plast Reconstr Aesthet Surg 2012;65(12):e366–7.
226. Murata K, Inada Y, Fukui A, et al. Clinical application of the reversed pedicled venous flap containing perivenous areolar tissue and/or nerve in the hand. Br J Plast Surg 2001;54(7):615–20.
227. Akita S, Kuroki T, Yoshimoto S, et al. Reconstruction of a fingertip with a thenar perforator island flap. J Plast Surg Hand Surg 2011;45(6):294–9.
228. Omokawa S, Yajima H, Inada Y, et al. A reverse ulnar hypothenar flap for finger reconstruction. Plast Reconstr Surg 2000;106(4):828–33.
229. Omokawa S, Takaoka T, Shigematsu K, et al. Reverse-flow island flap from the thenar area of the hand. J Reconstr Microsurg 2002;18(8): 659–63.
230. Omokawa S, Fujitani R, Dohi Y, et al. Reverse Midpalmar Island flap transfer for fingertip reconstruction. J Reconstr Microsurg 2009;25(3):171–80.
231. Orbay JL, Rosen JG, Khouri RK, et al. The glabrous palmar flap. Tech Hand Up Extrem Surg 2009; 13(3):145–50.
232. Pan XG, Tian WC, Guan TX. A clinical study on the extended reverse digital artery island flap. Zhonghua Zheng Xing Wai Ke Za Zhi 2004;20(1):33–4 [in Chinese].
233. Seyhan T. Reverse thenar perforator flap for volar hand reconstruction. J Plast Reconstr Aesthet Surg 2009;62(10):1309–16.
234. Hao PD, Zhuang YH, Zheng HP, et al. The ulnar palmar perforator flap: anatomical study and clinical application. J Plast Reconstr Aesthet Surg 2014;67(5):600–6.
235. Tapan M, İğde M, Yıldırım AR, et al. Hypothenar island flap: a safe and excellent choice for little finger defects. Indian J Plast Surg 2015;48(3):288–92.
236. Atasoy E, Ioakimidis E, Kasdan ML, et al. Reconstruction of the amputated finger tip with a triangular volar flap. A new surgical procedure. J Bone Joint Surg Am 1970;52(5):921–6.
237. Diaz LC, Vergara-Amador E, Fuentes Losada LM. Double V-Y flap to cover the fingertip injury: new technique and cases. Tech Hand Up Extrem Surg 2016;20(4):133–6.
238. Frandsen PA. V-Y plasty as treatment of finger tip amputations. Acta Orthop Scand 1978;49(3): 255–9.
239. Zhou X, Wang L, Mi J, et al. Thumb fingertip reconstruction with palmar V-Y flaps combined with bone and nail bed grafts following amputation. Arch Orthop Trauma Surg 2015;135(4):589–94.
240. Braga-Silva J, Gehlen D, Bervian F, et al. Randomized prospective study comparing reverse and direct flow island flaps in digital pulp reconstruction of the fingers. Plast Reconstr Surg 2009;124(6): 2012–8.
241. Chung KC, Hamill JB, Walters MR, et al. The Michigan Hand Outcomes Questionnaire (MHQ): assessment of responsiveness to clinical change. Ann Plast Surg 1999;42(6):619–22.
242. Stokvis A, Ruijs A, Neck J, et al. Cold intolerance in surgically treated neuroma patients: a prospective follow-up Study. J Hand Surg Am 2009;34(9): 1689–95.
243. Farzad M, Asgari A, Dashab F, et al. Does disability correlate with impairment after hand injury? Clin Orthop Relat Res 2015;473(11):3470–6.

Printed and bound by CPI Group (UK) Ltd, Croydon, CR0 4YY
03/10/2024
01040372-0008